Bi - Polar*oïd*

David Samuelson

Copyright © 2020 by David Samuelson.

Library of Congress Control Number:	2020900654
ISBN: Hardcover	978-1-7960-8275-3
Softcover	978-1-7960-8274-6
eBook	978-1-7960-8287-6

All rights reserved. No part of this book may be reproduced or transmitted in any form or by any means, electronic or mechanical, including photocopying, recording, or by any information storage and retrieval system, without permission in writing from the copyright owner.

Any people depicted in stock imagery provided by Getty Images are models, and such images are being used for illustrative purposes only.
Certain stock imagery © Getty Images.

Print information available on the last page.

Rev. date: 06/11/2020

To order additional copies of this book, contact:
Xlibris
1-888-795-4274
www.Xlibris.com
Orders@Xlibris.com
808267

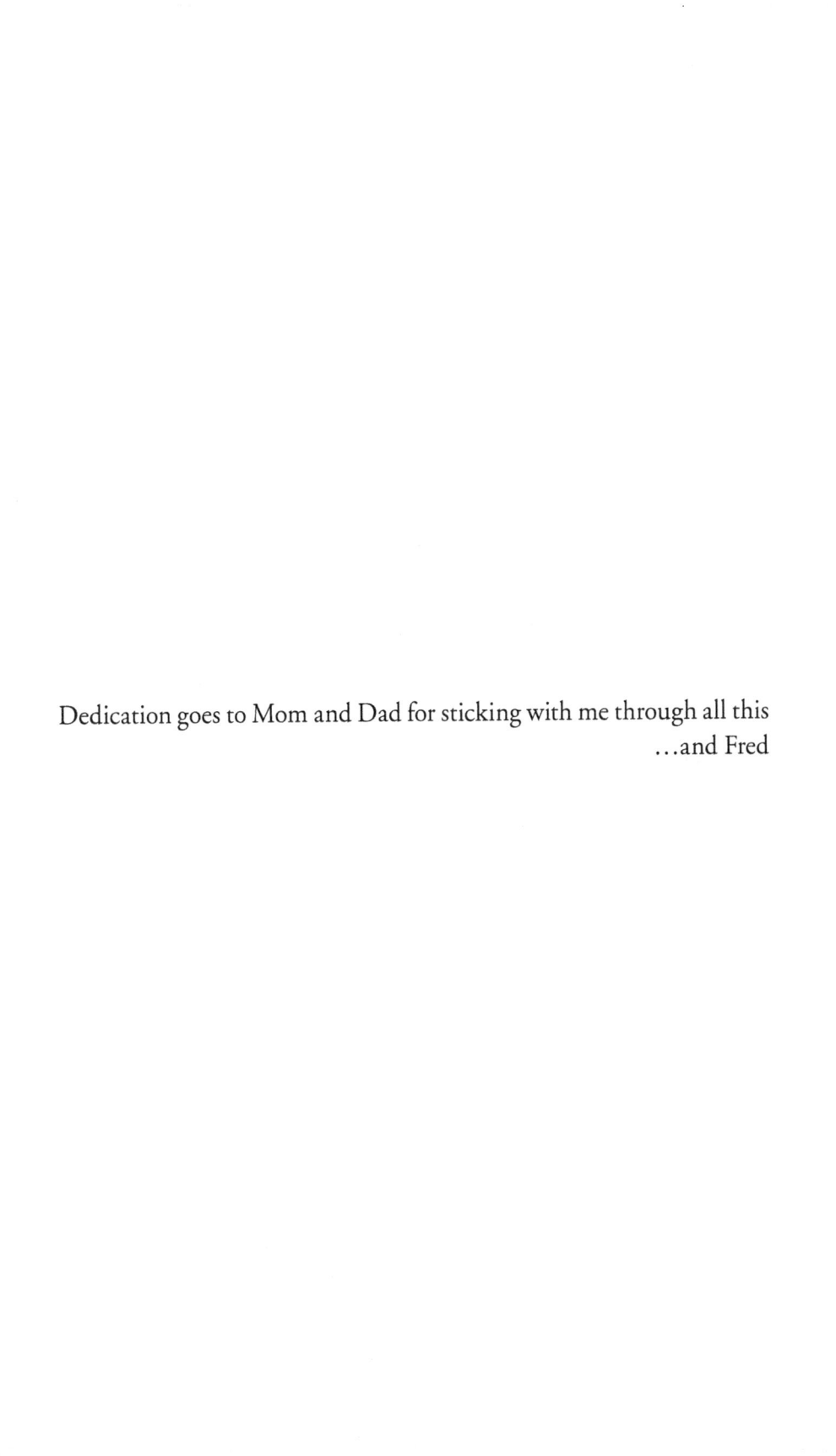

Dedication goes to Mom and Dad for sticking with me through all this
...and Fred

TABLE OF CONTENTS

Introduction v

Chapter 1: Michael Reese 1

Chapter 2: Somewhere Just North Of Capernicus 48

Chapter 3: Second Chance 62

Chapter 4: (Eighteen and over only - X rated) 78

Chapter 5: (Eighteen and over only - X rated) 85

Chapter 6: My World of Work - Post Pop-In - Renaissance Man ... 89

Chapter 7: 5/3/95 - Tammy's words on the answering machine ... 117

Chapter 8: Rockford - Hospital Stay - 1999 147

Chapter 9: The Present 183

Introduction

June 6, 1974

Why do people get depressed?
There are many reasons, nonetheless.
Some people lose confidence in themselves.
Others lose confidence in what they've done.
Still others lose confidence in their futures.
These are all the uncertainties of life;
What will happen, has happened, and is happening.
But, the most important thing to know,
Is the knowledge that life goes on no matter what.
Sure, life has its ups and downs,
But, you can't enjoy the good times,
If you want to end it all when things go bad.
So, take a tip from someone who knows.
Enjoy life while it's here.
And when depression starts to show its hand,
You have to work harder than ever to gain back what you had.

My Letter to Zelle

December 30, 2008

David: HONEY I AM HERE FOR YOU!!!

David: DID I TELL YOU MY PEN NAME?

David: DAVID SAMUELSON AND IF YOU DON'T CALL ME BACK, I WILL GO STRAIGHT TO THE PRINTERS TO GET COPIES FOR EVERYONE COMING TO OUR WEDDING. I KNOW YOU ARE MAD AT ME, BUT I TALKED TO MICHAEL JORDAN FOR AN HOUR ON SUNDAY EVENING. AND I HAVE NOT SHOWN ANYONE MY BODY, EVEN YOU!!!!! I DON'T PLAY WITH THAT STUFF. SO IF YOU DON'T WANT TO TALK TO ME NOW, I HAVE A LOT TO TAKE CARE OF TODAY. PASSPORTS, VISAS, MARRIAGE LICENSE, NEW CAR AND I NEED TO START LOOKING FOR A FURNISHED HOUSE FOR US IN THE WARRENVILLE AREA. I PROMISE YOU IF YOU DON'T SHOW YOUR FACE RIGHT NOW, I AM LEAVING AND THERE GOES YOUR TICKET TO THE PRESIDENTIAL INAUGURATION!!!

David: OH, BY THE WAY, DID I TELL YOU THAT I ORDERED OUR FAMILY CREST. IT IS THE ZELLE CREST FROM BAVARIA!!!

David: ALSO, ON CHRISTMAS EVE, YOU INSPIRED ME TO FINISH MY FIRST SONG WHICH WILL BE PERFORMED BY MY FIRST BAND FOR THE FIRST TIME ANYWHERE. IT WILL BE TELEVISED WORLDWIDE, BECAUSE IT IS A PART OF THE PRESIDENTIAL INAUGURATION WHICH I AM HOSTING.

David: THE BAND IS CALLED WWIII; WORLD WAR THREE. IT WILL INCLUDE MEMBERS OF AMERICA, JEFF LYNNE BEV BEVAN AND ROY WOOD FROM THE ELECTRIC LIGHT ORCHESTRA JUST TO NAME A FEW. I WILL BE THE LEAD SINGER AND MY PARTNERS AND FORMER BOSS FROM WHOLE FOODS MAKE UP THE BALANCE OF THE BAND. ALL PROCEEDS FROM THE SALE OF THE SINGLE WILL BE DONATED TO THE NATIONAL ALLIANCE FOR THE MENTALLY ILL AND THE DEPRESSION BIPOLAR SUPPORT ALLIANCE. I WILL ALSO BE PLAYING GUITAR WHICH I HAVE TAKEN LESSONS FOR OVER 7 YEARS. THERE WILL ALSO BE A SONG PERFORMED BY THE LEAD GUITARIST OF THE TINA TURNER BAND CALLED "ZELLE". YOU BRING OUT THE BEST IN ME HONEY. I COULD NEVER DO WITHOUT YOUR SUPPORT. I LOVE YOU SO VERY VERY MUCH.

David: BY THE WAY, I HAVE ALREADY RENTED OUT THE HOUSE THAT I LIVE IN RIGHT NOW, SO WE CAN MOVE INTO OUR NEW HOUSE WHEN WE CAN FIND IT.

Chapter 1

Michael Reese

Setting

A mental hospital in Chicago

Time

Monday night in late December

Scenery

Typical "One Flew over the Cuckoo's Nest"

Characters

Melissa
Donna
Dave
Mike
Tom
Gail
Lee
and various aides
Ruth
Dr. Levy

ACT 1

Scene 1

(The hospital is quiet and the P.P.I. is full except for the bed reserved for Dave. Dave and Lee and Ruth walk in the door)

Ruth: Where is the washroom?
Dave: How should I know?
Lee: Go look for it, you want me to hold your hand?

(This kind of discussion continues for about a half-hour until he is brought upstairs)

Scene 2

(The hospital ward at nine o'clock)

Dave: Hello everybody. My name is Dave.
Everybody: Hello Dave, my name is Se....(everybody's name said together).

(He was put in a room with Tom who made funny faces every time he looked Dave's way)

Dave: Hello Tom.

Tom: Hi.
Dave: Well, I guess I'll get to know some people a little better.
Tom: I don't care.

Dave: Okay, I'll see you later.

(He walked out into the day room. Then he saw her for the first time. Melissa walked in her robe looking better than a summer day. Dave fell in love instantly.)

(The night went on much as expected although Dave is much friendlier to the patients than they are to him. He needs a pill to fall asleep and afterward sleeps for five hours.)

Scene 3

(the next morning)

(Breakfast came at about 8:15 and it was very good. Mary and George sit with him.)

Dave: Well, if the food is this good every day, I won't mind staying here.
Mary: I don't like the food here. I eat much better at home.
George: I'm on a diet.
Dave: (looks up as Melissa walks into the room) Good morning Melissa.
Melissa: Good Morning.
Dave: How you feeling, okay?
Melissa: Yeh, I guess so.

(Dave finished his breakfast and went to sit next to Melissa.)

Dave: So what goes on here during the day?
Melissa: Not much, really.
Dave: Where are you from?
Melissa: I'm from Chicago.
Dave: Where in Chicago? I was brought up on the south side.

Melissa: On the south side, but I don't think it was anywhere near you.
Dave: And you're Jewish, right? (She nods her head) And we're both here. We seem to have a lot in common.
Melissa: I guess so, but so what?
Dave: Well at least I have someone to talk to.

(Melissa gets up and puts her tray away, then she goes to her room and gets dressed. Dave does the same only he goes to his room.)

(About a half-hour later)

Dave: Hi
Linda and Sue: Hi, Hi.
Dave: Hello again.

Dave and Gail

The love of my life,
Just happens to be my wife.
Although there has been much strife,
I think that it will be alright.
All my life I have had ups and downs.
It's like spinning around on a merry-go-round,
Because no matter where you go, you always come back,
With a hatred for man and a chip on your back.
Gail is just like a dream.
Although she has been having bad ones when I am depressed,
The prognosis is for sunny and warmer and we'll live happily ever after.

Melissa

The eyes are sincere and lovely,
But, not to look at bad things.
The hair is brown and beautiful,
But, not too long to cover good things.
The voice is sweet and pure,
But, not when it comes to unreal things.
The disposition is good and bad,
But, not to the point of no return.
The face is nice and pretty,
But, not when things displease her.
The ways of this woman please me,
But, how do I tell her how I feel?

Donna

Donna got the worst of it.
She always got punished.
Even though she wasn't that bad,
She always left our home.
She went away for self-preservation,
Until things would cool down and be somewhat normal.
I, in the meantime, would be counting my blessings,
That I was not Donna,
And not my sister.
Then she grew up and became a woman.
Although her title should be Mr. Clean,
And mine Mr. Obscene,
All things seem to be okay; calm and serene.
I LOVE YOU, DONNA.

Ernst

He's eighty, but not yet old.
He's beautiful and not yet wrinkled at all.
When Erna died he was more than bold,
And he took over for himself and did not stall.
He got his own place and refused to stay in the old one.
Even though he was lonely, he had his religion.
He had Steve and Debbie,
Donna and Dave,
Lee and Ruth
And thank God we have you!

The Lonely Old Man

The old man walked slowly up the stairs to his third floor apartment not knowing what time it was, nor caring. He was living alone since his wife had died and all he had were his two daughters, their husbands and their children; but it wasn't enough. He had become distraught in the last few days and his appetite had gone along with it.

He was a handsome man for his seventy-eight years. He had not shrunk hardly at all although his wife did before her untimely demise. He lived alone only because he liked to, and didn't want to be a burden on anybody. But, now he was lonely and he was ready to put an end to it all.

He opened his door with a start. Inside sat his wife next to his favorite chair. She was watching television and did not notice him come in. Then, strangely she fell asleep. The old man closed the door and opened it again. She was still there next to his favorite chair. He hurriedly turned off the T.V. as he did not want to wake his beautiful wife. He set out to make himself dinner. He felt good knowing that he could make two portions tonight since he had somebody to cook for. All of a sudden, sadness rushed over him again like a tidal wave on a beach. But, he shrugged it off since he felt this way very often. The dinner was definitely the best he had made in a long time. He sat down and starting eating his dinner. He didn't wake up his wife since he was sure that she was very, very tired. He finished eating both his portion and hers' and rubbed his fat belly and sighed a certain amount of relief. It was the first time that he had eaten well all week. Now he felt tired. He thought, well, I'll sleep before I turn on the television. The old man slowly picked up his cane and walked over to his favorite chair. He bent over and picked up a picture of his wife on a table next to his favorite chair. He kissed it and returned it to its resting place, promptly feeling even more relief. He sat down in his favorite chair and promptly went to sleep.

Sam

Fly away little Sam wherever you are,
Be you far away or very near.
My memory of you is everlasting.
Although, you were murdered in cold blood.
The clues in your death are still not clear.
The case is still open and the verdict is not in.
But, you were loved by the one that killed you.
May you rest in peace,
And steer clear of broken windows.

Amy

When you wake up in the morning,
With the sun just peeping its tired eye,
The furry animal named Amy bounds to attention.
White and black and brown and tan are her colors.
All of them clear and bright.
With eyes of brown, the darkest brown you've ever seen.
Even though the appearance is serene,
The actions are obscene.
I turn over on my back and look at the ceiling,
But, all that happens is the usual.
Amy gets the feeling that someone needs some healing.
Her tongue slips out both long and loving,
And it crosses my lips with love overflowing.
As I pause to close my eyes and open them,
I see my dog and think of Amy.

The Garbage

"Take out the garbage," said George's mother.

"I don't want to!"

"Do it, no complaints!"

"Alright, alright!"

George walked out into the cold winter and waded through foot deep snow. He opened the garage and saw an old man sitting on his car.

"Can I look through your garbage?" he said.

George was somewhat bewildered, but said yes anyway. The old man started eating the edible waste such as fat, bones, orange peels, potato peels and onion peels.

The old man sighed and said, "I've been eating garbage for two years now. You might say I am a human garbage disposal."

"Why did you start eating garbage?" asked George.

"I had no money for food so I had no choice."

"What does a potato peel taste like?"

"It tastes like a potato except it doesn't go down quite as easily."

George then shut the garage and went in out of the cold.

His mother said, "What took you so long?"

"I was eating the garbage."

"Oh, how was it?"

"It was alright except I've got to watch my weight. All that fat has a lot of calories."

George went upstairs and went to sleep. The next morning, he woke up and had an urge for an orange peel. He threw away the orange and ate the orange peel. It was alright and supposedly healthy.

That night the old man was in the garage again and looked at the garbage George brought out. The old man said. "I see you've been eating the normal waste. It works every time. This way I get to eat all the normal food."

Coco

Coco is a dog that is beyond repute,
The most obnoxious one I have ever met.
Although she loves the hand that feeds her,
She still crawls and begs for special treatment.
Coco is black and white, but mostly black,
And that is because it covers her whole back.
I love Coco although you are old,
May you live forever and keep coming back.

It's Obscene

He woke up with a start and he felt the presence of another. Not knowing who or what it was he pretended to be asleep and he didn't move a muscle. He even tried to hold his breath.

Then he heard a voice. It said, "You are obscene, you will go to hell. You must change or you will not go to heaven and be with my master."

The man sat up with a start. He exclaimed, "How am I obscene?"

The voice replied, "You smoke too much, both cigarettes and marijuana, you have been mentally ill and you drink too much,"

The man said, "But I can't stop, it is a part of my life, What can I do?"

The messenger said, "The only way to save yourself is to quit smoking, both cigarettes and marijuana, quit drinking, straighten your head out and stop having lude sexual affairs."

The man looked at himself in his mirror on the ceiling and said, "I'm sorry I cannot do anything of the sort. I am happy with my life and if I am forced to go to hell because of these normal things than I must."

Being rebuffed again the messenger of the devil left in a huff and man went back to sleep very pleased with himself.

I Love Everybody

To love and not to be loved back,
Is worse than being stabbed in the back.
You want to give so much,
But, she says forget you, go get some lunch.
Why is love so hard to communicate,
When the feeling is so real to me?
Why can't people love who they want to,
Without the approval of that person?
Love is a desire not a need,
So, why can't we all love each other,
And begin to do that and by that method,
Happiness and health will follow in time.

Waiting

Waiting ain't easy no matter how you slice it.
It's like a race horse chomping on the bit.
Sometimes I can't stand it, I have to wait so long.
Sometimes I even stop myself to take a bong.
Waiting in line is worst of all,
Because I could be home with my wife having a ball.
But waiting is necessary nonetheless,
If I could only calm myself and got some rest.

Scene 4
(that afternoon)

Scene 4 (that afternoon)
(Melissa and Dave are sitting alone in Melissa's room)

Dave: I notice you wear a cross. Why?

Melissa: I believe in Jesus. If we believe in other miracles of G-d, why not this one, too?

Dave: That's funny because I feel about the same way. I even watched a midnight mass on T.V. There's too many coincidences going on here. It's almost scary.

Melissa: No, it's not scary it's just coincidental. (Melissa gets up and Dave follows. Dave goes to his room and writes two poems, Amy and Melissa. After he writes it, he wants to read it to Melissa. So he asks her to come down to his room).

Dave: Here is the poem, I hope you enjoy it.

Melissa: All I want to know is how other people see me. (She reads the poem). I like it, it shows a lot of insight into my being. Do you mind if I show it to my doctor?

Dave: No, I'd be honored! And as time goes along I'll add to the poem. I'll make you a copy of it.

Melissa: Great!

(Dave retires to his room alone and rewrites it up quickly. He gives it to Melissa and she shows him how she feels by the expression on her face). (After this, Dave goes over to talk to his therapist since his feelings for Melissa and his wife are clashing. The lights fade out on this scene).

Act II
(The next day)
Scene 1

ACT 3

Scene 1

(Dave wakes up at 1:30 and starts to talk to one of the aides about his book. The aide likes his stories and poems and then Dave sets out to write this play. On the way to walking to his room, he notices Melissa sitting in the love seat).

Dave: Good night, Melissa.
Melissa: You are a hypocrite. You called me malicious.
Dave: No, I didn't. I called you Melissa.
Melissa: I don't believe you.
Dave: I don't expect you to. The more I say these days, the more you don't listen.
Melissa: And I don't want to hear anymore from you now.
Dave: Okay, I can appreciate you, but I still think a hell of a lot of you.

(Dave walked away then and down to his room. Then he walks back to talk to Melissa again).

Dave: Can I say one more thing?
Melissa: You've already said too much. You talk too much. (That last sentence, Dave joined her on it).

(Dave then went back to his room and got a yellow pad to write this play on).

(He started with scene 1 and scene 2 and then . . .)

Dave:	Do you mind if I move the television towards me a little bit?
Melissa:	No.
Dave:	what?
Melissa:	No!
Dave:	I think I need a hearing aide. So you really think I am malicious, huh?
Melissa:	I didn't say that.
Dave:	But you said that I was a hypocrite.
Melissa:	You are and not only that you have a big mouth.
Dave:	You really are malicious aren't you.

Melissa (raising her voice): You sure do talk a lot, don't you? (The nurse appears at the door of the nursing station).

Sheri:	What is going on out here?
Melissa:	He won't shut up.
Sheri:	Please keep your voices down.

(The nurse goes back into the office).

Dave:	You sure do show a lot of hatred don't you.
Melissa:	(She goes over to the nursing station and communicates with Sheri). (Sheri appears at the door).
Sheri:	Melissa is trying to listen to the T.V. Dave, please keep it down.
Dave:	So am I.
Sheri:	Okay.

(Twenty seconds pass as Dave looks at Melissa and Melissa looks at the wall).

Dave: I'm sorry.

(Then Dave goes back to writing and during this Melissa gets up and goes to bed. Dave waves at her and continues writing).

Hatred

I have the feeling that someone hates me.
Why, I don't know, but she has hurt me.
She doesn't know and doesn't even seem to care.
She's trying to be cold for some uncertain reason which she won't tell.
It's like having a dictionary and not knowing how to spell.
I hate being hated, it's a terrible feeling,
But, although I am hurt, my feelings are starting to heal.
I don't understand it and maybe I shouldn't care,
But, even though I really do care,
My heart and my brain have to be separate,
Or my understanding of myself will leave,
And if that happens, I lose my opportunity to believe!
P.S. She really does hate me!

Hurt

I am suffering right now for something I didn't do,
Because I happened to befriend someone who doesn't feel
she needs them.
And I don't know how to take it,
Whether to let the hurt show or cover it up with giggles and smiles.
I guess I'll never know the proper thing to do.
Because no one seems to know anymore than me,
Although their position says that they should.
Why this has happened to me, I will never know,
But I guess that fate tells us the time has come to lay off.
Even though I can't believe that it is true,
The answer is that no matter how I tried to please someone,
All I did is find out that no matter what I do,
This person will hate me and not like me.
I think I feel sorry for myself,
That's a strange thing to do considering I met her two days ago.
She's kind and sweet to everyone but me,
And I can't seem to figure it out,
Maybe it's me, maybe it's her.
Whomever it is, I am hurting.

Bob says . . .

He who tells lies, only ends up lying to himself.

Hurt is something to try to commumnicate to others.

Love means the understanding and compassion to forgive.

Melissa hates me.

I think I'm in love.

Writing is the best way to communicate when talking is too uncomfortable.

Television is only good when there is nothing better to do.

Radio is the entertainment capital.

Movies tell us about ourselves through other people's lives.

The president is the strongest, yet the weakest man in the nation.

Stubborness is the root of all evil.

Sports show just how dumb our idols can be.

Movie stars are just as human as we are. They have just been in the right place at the right time.

Eating

We are what we eat said the fat man to the short.
If only Berman and Lovell had known their fate,
They would have surely decided to abort.
But since they didn't, the only solution was we are what we eat.
When Columbus discovered America, the first thing he did,
Was to sample the food on this new place.
And because Columbus decided, we are what we eat,
He kept on eating and fell asleep.
When he awoke he awoke with a start,
Because he found himself fat and big,
Even though he had only eaten corn,
He was fat like a pig and he needed a shoe horn,
To get him back on his ship.
He was unsuccessful in getting on the Nina, the Pinta, or the SantaMaria.
One of his crew mates said, "how did you get so fat?"
I don't know, he said, all I did was eat ten whole ears of corn!

Sleep

I need some coffee, I have to wake up,
My doctor is coming at seven-o'clock.
The coffee isn't ready so I'll write this poem,
And fall asleep writing about jogging around the block.
My coffee is here, thank the Lord,
If only I could feel as sleepy when it's time to go to sleep.

Here's Johnny

"Here's Johnny", said Ed McMahon,
With Doc bowing his spindly body at the star of the show.
The monologue was not funny as usual,
But, Mr. Carson found a way to make it funny.
His guests tonight included John Wayne, Red Skelton, and David Samuelson.
The audience laughed at the last two names,
But, Red and David did not feel bad,
Since their jobs are to entertain the audience.
The laughter pleased the two performers.
Red was successful and so was John Wayne,
And, now it was time for me to appear.
And then, I threw up off stage and came on white and weak.
Then Johnny said, "You look good, how are you?"
I realized the makeup had covered up the incident.
And Johnny, and the audience and me lived happily after.

The First Jewish President

The T. V. was on and no one was listening. He so wanted the public to listen to his speech. He wanted to be the president of the United States. The world had changed and had become strongly overpopulated. Congress had passed a law and it was up to the president to sign the bill into law. The law stated that all mentally-retarded children would be put to death upon birth to save the government money and to promote the PGAS, the population growth appreciation society.

Time passed and Mr. Cohn became our first Jewish president. And not only that, his daughter Joy got married to the nicest young man she had ever met. Mr. Cohn was so happy that he couldn't believe that all that was happening was really happening. There could only be one thing that could make him happier and that would be a grandson. Then it happened. Joy became pregnant and was expecting in seven months. The nation was preparing for the child too, since President Cohn was the most popular president since Kennedy.

And then it happened. The president's grandson was born and it became evident right away that he was mongoloid. The President and his wife, their daughter and her husband were distraught. The only person not upset by it was the son of the President. He was very liberal and wanted the baby put to death. The President then went into action. The President gave the doctor a thousand dollar bill. The doctor then marked on the birth certificate that the baby was normal not mentally retarded. At first Joy was overjoyed that her son would be given the opportunity to live. Later on she became very depressed. And she got to the point where she wanted to kill the baby. Then one day she put the baby in a trash compactor and turned it on. All of a sudden, she felt a wave of relief. Then she went on television and stated what her father had done. Impeachment proceedings started immediately. They were unsuccessful, but he lost his favor with his family, friends, public and not only that, the next election, he lost his job. The next year, he died of old age at the age of sixty.

Divorce

And now it's time to end the relationship,
Although the past two and a half years haven't been all
that bad,
She doesn't want to give it another try,
Even though I have changed my evil ways.
Right now I am at Reese and am getting help.
She is living with her sister and nephew,
And taking care of a five month old child.
I just want her to learn how to take care of herself,
While I am doing the same in a conducive situation.
She won't believe me no matter what I say,
So what can I do but end it for self-preservation.
Too bad it has to happen, but that's the way the ball bounces.
I wish her health and happiness and all the knowledge in the
world.
Hopefully I will find the same some day!

Loneliness

People leave you alone, there's no one to talk to.
You feel alone and that nobody cares.
What do you do? You occupy yourself with anything,
From playing cards to talking on the phone.
Doing these things makes you feel like you're really not
alone.
But sometimes your so lonely, you feel like a piece of stone,
And no matter what you do, you feel as cold as a bone.
The only thing to do is to try and make believe you are somewhere else,
In a different climate with a bunch of people.
It's hard to do sometimes, closing you eyes helps,
Listening to music also helps, although those things can't replace the emptiness in your heart.
Grin and bear it is the answer because things could only get better.

Bob says . . .

A thought unspoken is a thought that might as well have not been thought.

Overpopulation and the bomb will kill us before man kills himself.

Doctors and nurses only take care of you when they have the time.

Melissa went to the dentist.

Fire and water go together like love and sex.

Christmas and New Years are either the happiest or saddest holidays of the year.

Chairs are for sitting, seats are for shitting.

Music says it all.

I love you Harry.

Hot Chocolate reminds me of cannibalism.

Roses are red

Violets are blue

If I don't get out of here soon

I will blow up like a balloon.

THE SAVIOR

THE MAN WAS FRAIL AND WEAK WITH A TALL, LANKY BODY. HE DID NOT HAVE MANY FRIENDS, ALTHOUGH, HE WAS PLEASANT TO BE AROUND. ONE DAY THE MAN WAS SITTING ON A PARK BENCH MINDING HIS OWN BUSINESS, WHEN A MUGGER APPROACHED HIM WITH A GUN AND DEMANDED HIS MONEY.

THE MAN SAID, "I HAVE NOTHING OF VALUE, BUT MY LIFE. TAKE THAT AND I WILL SURELY HAVE NOTHING."

THE MUGGER DIDN'T BELIEVE HIM OF COURSE AND TOOK HIS WALLET. HE OPENED IT AND ALL THAT CAME OUT OF IT WAS BIRD SEED. THE ROBBER WAS GETTING MAD NOW AND SAID, "HOW DID YOU GET HERE TODAY!?"

"I WALKED FROM MY APARTMENT," SAID THE MAN.

"OKAY," SAID THE MUGGER, "LET'S GO SEE WHAT YOU HAVE IN THERE."

IT WAS A SHORT WALK TO THE MAN'S APARTMENT. THEY WENT IN AND SAW A MIRACULOUS THING. STANDING IN THE MIDDLE OF THE FLOOR WAS A GIANT CRUCIFIX. THE PLACE WAS EMPTY BESIDES THAT.

THE MUGGER SPOKE, "IS THIS SOME SORT OF A JOKE?"

"NO," SAID THE MAN, "I SLEEP ON THE FLOOR AND I EAT OUT."

"WHAT DO YOU PAY FOR YOUR FOOD WITH?"

"I WORK FOR MY DAILY BREAD," SAID THE MAN GETTING RATHER UPSET HIMSELF.

THE MUGGER LOOKED AT THE CRUCIFIX AND NOTICED THAT THE CROSS WAS MADE OF THE FINEST WOOD. HE DECIDED TO TAKE IT. HE NO SOONER PICKED IT UP WHEN HE WAS TRANSPORTED BACK TO JESUS'S TIME AND WAS PROMPTLY CRUCIFIED.

THE MAN THEN SAID OUT LOUD, "WHY DO PEOPLE HAVE TO KEEP BOTHERING ME? I DO NOTHING TO

PROVOKE THEM. G-D, GIVE ME THE STRENGTH TO CARRY ON."

IT WAS GETTING LATE, THEN, AND TIME TO SLEEP. THE MAN WORE GLOVES AND SHOES ALL THE TIME, EVEN TO SLEEP. THIS MADE HIM A LITTLE ECCENTRIC, BUT PEOPLE WOULD START TO WONDER IF THEY SAW THE HOLES IN HIS HANDS AND FEET.

THE BEDTIME STORY

THERE ONCE WAS A MAN NAMED BOB AND A GIRL NAMED MELISSA. THEY LIVED IN A THREE BEDROOM HOME WITH AMY, THEIR PARROT. BOB WAS AN ENCYCLOPEDIA SALESMAN BY TRADE AND MELISSA WAS AN AVON LADY. THE HAPPINESS THEY ENJOYED SPRANG FROM THEIR LIVES LIKE A BABBLING BROOK.

THEN ONE DAY, MELISSA CAME HOME FROM SELLING TO SAY SHE FELT NAUSEOUS. SHE DECIDED TO GO TO A DOCTOR. THE DOCTOR SAID THAT SHE WAS PREGNANT. MELISSA WAS OVERJOYED AND SHE TOLD BOB AS SOON AS HE GOT HOME. BOB WAS VERY HAPPY AND DECIDED TO HAVE A PARTY IN TWO WEEKS.

TWO WEEKS LATER, EVERYBODY AND THEIR BROTHER-IN-LAW SHOWED UP. SUDDENLY, IT WAS OBVIOUS THAT ONE OF THE PEOPLE WAS NOT THEIR FRIEND. AS SOON AS MELISSA PICKED UP THE TELEPHONE TO CALL THE POLICE, THE UNFRIENDLY MAN APPROACHED HER WITH A GUN. MELISSA PUT UP HER HANDS AND SCREAMED. THE PARTY HALTED AND EVERYBODY JUMPED ON THE MAN AT ONCE. THEN, THERE WAS A SHOT AND A HIGH SHRILL SCREAM. MELISSA FELL OUT OF THE PILE WITH A THUD. SHE WAS SHOT IN THE STOMACH. THE BABY DIED IMMEDIATELY AND MELISSA WAS VERY SAD. BUT, BOB SAID, "AT LEAST WE HAVE EACH OTHER."

THE BULLET DID NOT EFFECT HER FROM HAVING ANOTHER CHILD. BOB AND MELISSA HAD TWO LOVELY CHILDREN, A BOY AND A GIRL. THEY NEVER HAD ANOTHER PARTY. MELISSA AND BOB LIVED HAPPILY EVER AFTER EXCEPT FOR ONE THING. THEIR GRANDMOTHER DIED THAT YEAR AND SADDENED THE FAMILY, BUT THOSE KIND OF THINGS DO HAPPEN. THEIR GRANDFATHER LIVED TO A RIPE OLD AGE AND LIVED HAPPILY EVER AFTER.

DOUBLE STANDARD

ONE DAY, LEE WANTED TO DO SOMETHING, NOTHING IMPORTANT, JUST GO OUTSIDE AND PLAY SOFTBALL. HIS MOTHER SAID YOU HAVE TO CHANGE YOUR CLOTHES BEFORE YOU GO OUT. HE DID IT AND WENT OUT TO PLAY.

AT ABOUT 6:00 P.M., HIS MOTHER YELLED, "LEE, DINNER!" LEE OBEDIENTLY CAME IN TO EAT DINNER. LATER, HE WANTED TO WATCH TELEVISION SO HE ASKED HIS MOTHER. SHE SAID, "YES." LATER SHE SAID, "LEE, IT'S TIME FOR BED." LEE JUMPED TO ATTENTION AND WENT TO BED.

THE NEXT DAY WAS SATURDAY AND LEE WANTED TO GO SHOPPING. "MOM, CAN WE GO SHOPPING?"

"NO," SAID HIS MOTHER, "I HAVE OTHER THINGS TO DO."

JUST THEN HIS FATHER CAME HOME. HE SAID, "HELLO LEE. HAVE YOU MADE A DECISION ON WHAT YOU WANT TO DO WITH YOUR EDUCATION? YOU HAVE A CHOICE OF GOING AWAY TO SCHOOL OR I'LL BUY YOU A CAR AND YOU WILL GO TO SCHOOL AROUND HERE. WHAT WOULD YOU LIKE TO DO?"

LEE SAID, "I WANT TO GO AWAY!" HE DIDN'T BOTHER TELLING THEM WHY. HE DIDN'T WANT TO HURT THEIR FEELINGS, BUT, HE COULDN'T STAND LIVING WITH THEM ANYMORE. "DAD, YOU WANT TO GO SHOPPING?"

"NO, SON, I'M TOO TIRED."

"CAN I TAKE YOUR CAR AND GO BY MYSELF?"

"NO, I'M SORRY YOU CAN'T."

"CAN I TAKE YOUR CAR, MOM?"

"NO, I DON'T LIKE THE WAY YOU DRIVE!"

"WELL, YOU WON'T BE DRIVING WITH ME!"

DAD SAID, "PLEASE NO ARGUMENTS, I'VE HAD A HARD WEEK!"

LEE THEN WENT TO HIS ROOM TO WORK ON HIS JIGSAW PUZZLE. LEE THOUGHT ABOUT THE FACT THAT HE IS EXPECTED TO BE CALM WHILE JUMPING TO ATTENTION. WHY CAN'T THEY. OH WELL, I GUESS THAT'S THE WAY OF THE WORLD. HE THEN PUT THE NEXT PIECE IN HIS PUZZLE.

I Quit Smoking

Strike up the band, start marching, the celebration should begin.
I quit smoking cigarettes today for health reasons.
My lungs are black and my spirit is foggy,
But soon the smoke will be lifted from my life.
And probably I will love my wife of two years.
But that's life in the old tennis game of love.
I feel like running a mile in the nude,
or skinny dipping across the English Channel,
The only thing I'm allowed to do is to go to adjunctive therapy.
And play ping pong and sing and talk with beautiful adolescents.
Tomorrow is another day filled with football and excitement.
I pick Denver and Minnesota in the Championship games,
And Denver to win the Super Bowl.
My hat is off to Puff the Magic Dragon,
May he rest in peace and never may tar and nicotine touch my lungs again.

Skyhawk

It's blue and sleek with a hatchback.
It's fast and quick although it's doesn't show.
To take a girl in the car,
Is like spending a day at a bar.
The hatchback is the best feature of it all,
And there's enough room for a rendevous for two,
Or if you're kinky enough, for three.
The stick shift is on the floor,
Automatic not manual, I'm not that old.
If only it lasts as long as I want it to,
I will be eighty and my car sixty-two!

Sports

Baseball is the national pastime, but it's not my favorite.
Football is my favorite, but it's not the national pastime.
Golf is the dumbest game I know of.
You hit the ball cause you don't want it there,
But if you don't want it why do you chase after it?
Hockey is probably the most violent game,
Because it's so easy to get hurt or maimed.
Tennis is the best game for anyone to play to keep in shape.
Soccer is the up and coming sport where we kick a ball around.
It's an exciting game, but it will never be as popular as it
is in other countries.
Basketball is another one of my favorites.
It's fast paced and exciting.
I think all athletes get paid too much,
But that's my opinion and mine alone,
But since I don't sign their paychecks,
I really don't care.

Daddy's Dead

My daddy died last night driving on the highway.
He was my favorite daddy and a friend to the end.
His job was rigorous and everybody respected him.
Thank G-d for that or he'd still be a butcher.
Dakota Packing was the name of his company.
He had two partners Bob and Bert, both smart as whips,
And then there was Mike and Butch who were the best of all,
And then there was me, I worked long and hard, but not long enough.
My father needed me and now he's gone.
My mother and sister took it the hardest.
He was the man in their lives,
But life goes on anyway even though it's going to be nearly impossible.
Rest in peace and come back again, never leave again.
Be prepared to come to attention at any time because I need you, too.

The Dying Wish

Jim had just been in a terrible accident. He was in serious condition at a local hospital and the chances for him living were slight. He kept on murmuring, "Melissa, Melissa," so, she was summoned. When she arrived, Jim said to her, "Don't forget to take care of Amy!' And that was it. Jim was gone. He was buried two days later with a funeral very well attended.

Melissa went home and took care of Amy, the dog, and Melissa's life was well rewarded by it. Everytime she would leave Amy alone, the next morning she would feel ill. One day she was walking Amy, and as they crossed the street, a car struck Melissa. Amy ran away for help and came back with a police officer. Melissa was alright except for a minor concussion and a temporary case of amnesia. Amy, of course, did not understand this and started taking her vengeance out on Melissa.

Two days later, Melissa awoke and asked, "Where's Amy?" "We don't know", said her nurse. Melissa got out of the hospital shortly after that and knew where to find Amy. Melissa was physically sick and had to be confined to a wheel chair. When she got to Jim's grave site, there was Amy sitting in mourning of her dead master. Melissa said, "Amy, I'm back to take care of you." Amy ran into Melissa's arms, but the impact of the dog on Melissa's stomach caused internal bleeding. On her death bed Melissa said, "Kill that goddamn Amy, she's dangerous!"

Later that day Amy was put to death.

Moral: Always take care of those you care about only if the person knows why you are caring for them.

The Hair Dryer

Kevin stepped out of the shower with a wet head of hair. He took his hairdryer and turned it on. Nothing happened. He flipped it on and off a couple of times, but nothing. Being in a hurry he got mad and threw the hair dryer on the floor, Then it turned on and he dried his hair.

The next day, the same thing happened. This time he dropped the hair dryer and nothing happened. He dropped it again and it went on. This went on for a while until Kevin didn't have enough times to keep dropping it in order to get it to work, so he decided to buy a new hair dryer. No sooner did he say that, the hair dryer went on. He dried his hair and went to work.

The next day he took a shower and his hair dryer went on without him turning it on, but it went off before he was halfway through with drying his hair. No matter what he did, it would not go on. He then threw it in the incinerator.

The next day he did not have a hair dryer, so . . . he went out and bought one before he took a shower. He spent a little more money on this one and he was glad that he had. He ran a comb over his bald head and said, "I'm sure glad I've got a hair dryer that works!"

Holidays

Holidays are happy times for energy and cheer.
They are also sad times for those who have nobody.
Depression can set in and suicide can follow.
Numbers like suicide prevention aren't open all night,
So a lot of times things that could be prevented are not.
For those who have friends and family,
Holidays can be filled with dreams fulfilled.
And by surprises galore and much much more.
Too bad holidays can't be that way for everybody,
But to all I wish goodwill and may there be peace on earth.

Getting Out

It feels so good to almost be free.
I signed a five-day release yesterday,
And I feel very good about it.
The only bad thing is I can't get out for a week,
And I hope by then I am still able to speak.
I am getting angry very easily,
And that's because I'm ready to get out now.
The only thing is I can't and if it weren't for A.T.,
I'd be just as crazy as everybody else around here.
So I'll say farewell to this place with some fond memories.
I'll also have some sad memories,
But anyway you say it, it comes out the same.
I'm sure glad that I changed my name.

I WAS AN M.D. FROM BIRTH

Bob at 15

You know what? My voice finally changed and I'm even getting a few whiskers. The girls like me and I don't know why. There was a girl when I was a freshman who had a crush on me, but I couldn't respond so she dropped me. I was too shy. Then there was Jill and she thought an awful lot of me. Then she moved and all I was left with was memories and the five leaf clover she gave me. The guys didn't like me very much and they made fun of me constantly. I guess I wasn't as big and tough as they were. But I didn't care because I didn't want to be like them. I wanted to be myself, someone different, someone special, an individual, a leader. Then there was Steve and David who were both my best friends for a while. Then they both moved away. I was very sad because that always seemed to happen. I guess I am feeling sorry for myself again. But I think I deserve to. I had an unhappy high school life. I appeared in plays and became people I would like to be like. Thank G-d for my acting ability and my musical talents. Too bad I can't write worth a darn!

A Fairy Fable

Once upon a time, there lived a man named David. He had a wife named Amy and a cat named Sam. One day, David came home from his construction job and said that he had to quit his job because of a fight he had with his boss. He was very depressed and so were Amy and Sam. David decided he wasn't going to sit on his laurels so he went over to his piano and started playing.

Amy and Sam were very surprised considering David had never played piano. What he played sounded good but it sounded hollow and unreal to the ear. Amy sat down and picked up David's guitar and started playing along with him.

David and Sam were very surprised considering Amy had never played guitar. Sam got up from his bed and said in a very loud voice, "Well, if you two are going to play music, I'm going to have to find a job." The cat moved towards the door and jumped through her crawl space. Two hours later, Sam came back saying that no one wanted a talking cat because he didn't have any schooling.

Sam then started to cry. Amy got up from her chair and exclaimed, "Well, if Sam can't get a job and David is still playing piano, then I have to go out and look for a job."

Three hours later, Amy returned and exclaimed, "I can't find a job because they say I have to have graduated college!" Amy then started to cry.

David finally got up from his piano and exclaimed, "Since both of you can't find a job, I'll have to look for a job myself!"

One hour later, David returned with tears in his eyes. Amy and Sam looked at him and knew he couldn't find a job. All of a sudden, a fairy godfather appeared and said, "I'll grant everyone of you one wish."

Amy said, "I want a college diploma." She got it. Sam said that he wanted some catnip and he got it. David sat still for a while and said, "I have everything I want. I have Amy and Sam, the two people I love: what more could I want?"

The fairy godfather looked perplexed and said, "I can not leave until I grant you a wish."

"Okay," said David, "then go out and find a job and support us for the rest of our lives!"

The fairy godfather then left and found a job, supported the family and became very unhappy. One day, the fairy godfather approached David and said, "I can't stand working construction. If I give you one more wish, will you allow me to leave?"

David thought for a moment and said, "Okay, I have a kind heart, but let me think about what I want to wish for." An hour later, after much discussion and fighting with both Amy and Sam, David exclaimed, "I want to be the richest man in the world!"

The fairy godfather snapped his fingers and then disappeared. All of a sudden, gold started to fall from the sky and David became very, very happy.

At the same time, Amy, who had been getting bored with playing the guitar, decided to go out and get a job. She left and she never came back.

Sam then said, "I am going to find a female cat. I want a family!" Sam left and he never came back.

David, forever mourning the loss of Amy and Sam, lived alone for the rest of his life.

Moral: Riches are only in the eye of the beholder! Sometimes you have more before you have anything at all.

The End

The Chocolate Bar

Dennis ran outside with true abandon to play football. The only thing was that none of his friends wanted him on their team. Dennis didn't care, though, because every once in a while, he'd surprise everybody and make a good play.

It was getting dark now and he knew it was time for dinner. He ran home and into the house. He snuck into the candy drawer and pulled out a chocolate bar. He ate it quickly and then threw away the wrapper before his mother came into the room. His mother knew that he got diarrhea whenever he ate chocolate, but he loved it so much that he ate it anyway. It was also a reward for himself since he made such a good play today.

He went to sleep early that night and woke up the next morning with a very strange feeling. He felt taller some how. He got up and looked in the mirror. He didn't recognize himself. He went downstairs and his mother took a double-take. She said that she wouldn't believe it if she weren't seeing it with her own two eyes. He was a foot taller and weighed 170 pounds.

He went to school that day and of course everybody treated him very strangely. He took it as admiration and went home from school happy for the first time in a long time.

He snuck a chocolate bar as he did the day before. All of a sudden he felt *very* strange. Not only did he grow a foot on the spot, but he also gained about fifty more pounds.

"Oh well," said Dennis out loud. "I wonder how Mom is going to take this!"

His mom walked in and gaped. Then she started to cry.

"What has happened to my son? First, he's shorter than everybody, now he's much taller!"

"Mom," said Dennis, "I like being tall!"

"Okay son, but be careful. Being seven feet tall will not be easy either!"

Dennis went over to the mirror and looked at himself. Then, he started to cry. "I want to be short again," said Dennis very sadly.

His mirror image replied, "You always wanted to be tall, now you've got your wish. Instead of complaining about it, you're going to have to try to be happy being tall just like you tried to make the most out of being short."

"Alright," said Dennis, "I guess I'll have to get used to it!"

Dennis made the best of being seven feet tall and became a star basketball player. He married a woman who was just slightly shorter than he was. His life was fairly happy, except he missed his chocolate bars. He was afraid of what would happen if he ate another bar.

Finally, though, fifty years after he ate his last chocolate bar, he decided to try one. He shrunk a foot and lost fifty pounds. Dennis and his wife were very unhappy since she was just under seven feet tall.

His wife said, "What are we going to do, Dennis?"

"I'm not sure," replied Dennis, "but maybe if you try some of this chocolate bar, you will shrink, too."

His wife decided to try some chocolate, but all she got was an acute case of diarrhea!

Chapter 2

Somewhere Just North Of Capernicus . . .

Romulus and Remus are sitting in the control room of their spaceship, Eagle. The Eagle is a quiet, maintenance free vessel allowing the pilots ample free time. They are playing a board game called, "Outer Space Invasion".

Romulus speaks. "I win again Remus. Maybe next time we play, you should try landing your ship before you disembark from it."

"Good idea, Romulus. By the way, which asteroid are we going to today?"

"One called Capernicus," retorts Romulus succinctly.

"I sure am hungry, Romulus. Can't we stop along the way and get a bite to eat?"

Romulus answers, "Our mission is to the asteroid Capernicus. Sometimes in life, Remus, we must be patient. Can you wait?"

"I suppose so," Remus replies sadly.

Three days later in the home of Ethel and Fred Cunningham . . .

"That saucer thing has been out there for three whole days. You gotta do something about that. I'm getting sick and tired of being cooped up in this goddamn house!"

"Ethel, what do you want me to do? I decide that I am going to go out and then you promptly talk me out of it. *Now*, you want me to go outside! What gives?!!"

Meanwhile . . .

Romulus looks at Remus and sighs. They are both thinking the same thing. This species is usually very hard to catch. It takes a battle of wits before we get together with them.

Back in the house . . .

Fred looks at his wife and says, "Why don't you go out there. Am I supposed to risk my life just because you are claustrophobic?"

Grandma sees what is happening and speaks. "Children, children! Why must you fight so much! When, Grandpa was alive, G-d rest his soul, we never fought. What is with you young whippersnappers?"

"Mother," says Fred, "we are all scared. Don't you think it's natural to get a little on edge?"

"No you children must learn to control yourselves!"

"Grandma," says Ethel, "let's calm down now, we are upsetting the child."

"You're not, upsetting me," says Debbie. "I see you guys fighting all the time. Besides that, I am sixteen you know!"

"No, your not sixteen. You won't be sixteen for two weeks," says Grandma.

"Goddamn it Grandma, I'm sick of you correcting me!"

"Just listen to that language, would you? You'd think by listening to her that she wasn't brought up right," defends Grandma.

Fred and Ethel, then, get mad at Grandma who promptly gets mad at Debbie when all of a sudden, they here a knock on the door. They all freeze and nobody says a word.

"It's the Avon lady," says Remus in his best falsetto voice.

"What do you think, Fred? Has an Avon lady ever lied to you?" whispers Ethel.

"Yes, but I can't tell you about it," says Fred with a snicker.

"What do you mean you can't tell me about it! I have a right to know. I am your wife, you know!"

"Oh, shove it Ethel!"

The knocking comes again.

"Oh Romulus, who did I say we were when I knocked before?" whispers Remus.

"Does that matter? What you should have said is that we are intergalactic visitors from another galaxy," replies Romulus.

Remus thinks for a moment, then says, "Hey let us in. We are friends from down the road a piece." (A big piece, says Remus under his breath.) "We are in trouble, help us."

"See Fred, it wasn't the Avon lady after all!"

Ethel walks over toward the door and opens it very slowly. Before she knows it there are two short beings standing behind her. Debbie begins screaming at the top of her lungs. Grandma fakes a faint, but she gets up when she realizes that everybody knows she is faking it. Fred just kind of smiles at the beings. Ethel, hearing all the commotion behind her decides not to turn around just yet. Then, she thinks better of it and makes a mad dash toward Fred.

Remus speaks first, "Hey, kid, shut up would you? Our ears are sensitive!"

Since Debbie is Debbie after all, she starts screaming at a much higher and louder pitch.

Remus, getting more nervous by the second, says, "How do we get her to close her mouth, Romulus?"

"Well, Remus," says Romulus calmly, "I am glad you asked that question. There are many different ways to quiet an acab. One way is to forcefully put your hand over their mouth. Another way is to hit them over the head with a dull object. Another is to wound the acab fatally."

"That is absolutely amazing, Romulus. Where did you learn that from?"

"Oh, I can't stand it, Remus."

"What's that Romulus?"

"I feel funny."

"What hurts?" exclaims Remus excitedly!

"No, no, I feel a joke coming on."

Debbie suddenly stops screaming and exclaims, "Finally, some entertainment!"

Romulus tells his joke. "Well remember you asked me how to quiet an acab and I told you. And then you asked me where I aquired that knowledge?"

Believe it or not, everybody is listening intently to Romulus; waiting impatiently for the punch line. They all say yes to Romulus' question.

"I learned about it on one of my many voyages through, The Twilight Zone," deadpans Romulus in his best Rod Serling.

Debbie and Remus begin laughing hysterically while the other three look at each other trying to figure out what is so funny. When the laughing subsides, Remus speaks to Debbie.

"What is your name?"

"Debbie, what's yours?"

"Remus, and this is Romulus. I have a question for you. How come you are so different from these older ones?"

"That is the older generation, (pointing at her parents and grandmother), and I am a part of the younger generation. I just can't seem to communicate with those old fogies!"

"On our asteroid," says Remus, "everybody is so old that all the generations seem to intertwine together."

Romulus, seeing the obvious sexual connotations in what Remus said, decides to stop the conversation when a sudden knock on the door does it for him.

"Open up Debbie, it's me, David."

Romulus looks at Remus and then speaks to Debbie. "Tell him to wait for you in his vehicle. No more!"

"David, wait in the car. I'll be out in a little while."

Romulus waits until he can no longer hear David's footsteps, then says, "Who is this David to you?"

"He is my boyfriend and I love him. We are going to get married someday."

Ethel speaks. "What do you mean you're going to marry David. You can do a lot better than that farm hand!"

"But, Mom, we're going to have our own farm someday. That is our dream. And anyway, why do you always have to give me such a hard time whenever I want to do anything."

"Because I'm your mother, that's why!"

"Both of you, stop arguing," interrupts Romulus.

They both cease abruptly.

"Now, Debbie," continues Romulus, "what your mother says makes no difference to me or to you. I like you and not only that, Remus loves you. So go to your David and never come back again. There is nothing for you here and there will be nothing for you here."

Remus interrupts Romulus and says, "I usually don't like to get serious, but maybe we should grade them before she goes."

"Good thinking, Remus. I know I had you along on this mission for some reason."

Romulus reaches into a pouch and takes out four medallions; one made of gold, one of silver, one of copper and one of solid lead.

"I think it is very obvious," says Romulus." The male is of primal quality, don't you think, Remus?"

Remus nods his head and then takes the gold medallion from Romulus and places it over Fred's head.

"Now, this is really a choice between Debbie and her mother, but, I think Debbie's mother is of better quality," says Romulus.

Debbie normally would have argued this point, but since she knows she is going to leave soon, she lets it pass. Her mother is gloating over her triumph. Remus then places the silver medallion over Ethel's head.

"Debbie is of good quality, though, so we will make her copper."

The medallion is placed over her head.

"You know, Romulus, that old one reminds me of the utility pipes back home. She's definitely lead, yeh, lead all the way."

The lead medallion is placed over her head amid harsh words.

"Now all of you, try to remove your medallions," insists Romulus.

They all try, but Debbie is the only one able to remove her copper label.

"Debbie, give me your medallion," says Romulus.

She does as she is told.

Remus, becoming very serious, says, "First, you may never tell anyone about us. If you do you will experience the consequences. Second, you are still young. Make something of yourself. And, also, try to make Capernicus an asteroid that you can be proud of.

"You mean Earth, don't you?" says Debbie shyly.

"Yes, child," says Remus, "now run along."

Debbie says a quick goodbye to her family and then looks at Romulus and Remus, smiles, and speaks. "I love you, too, Remus." Then she is out the door in a flash.

Ethel is crying by now and hanging on to Fred for dear life. Grandma is calm, but weak.

Romulus motions for the three acabs to follow them and they do so involuntarily since the medallions force them to follow. When they reach the ship, Remus rings the doorbell on the side of the craft.

A voice answers from inside, "Who's there?"

Romulus says, "It is Romulus and Remus and three acabs."

The voice replies, "What the hell is an acab?"

Remus says, "I don't know, just let us in!"

The door opens and the five of them file inside. Fred, Ethel and Grandma are taken to the recesses of the ship, while Romulus and Remus slip into the control room. The door closes behind them.

Remus can't stand it anymore. "What the hell is an acab?"

"I think I should call it the Romulan code. What I do is reverse the letters of a foreign word in order to cover up our intentions. But they can figure it out if they are smart enough."

"Where do, they speak the language that you used today?"

"Somewhere south of where we are today."

"I don't want to seem dumb, Romulus, but what does baca mean?"

"Cattle, Remus, cattle."

"Romulus, you are a genius!"

Just then there is a knock on the door. Romulus pushes a button and the door opens. It is one of the servants. He speaks. "What would you gents like for dinner tonight? Gold or silver?"

Romulus replies, "We will both take gold."

"Very well," says James. "By the way, that lead you brought in wasn't worth the trouble to catch her."

Remus interjects, "Don't throw the lead away. Make regrub out of her."

"What?" says James and leaves to put in the dinner order.

Romulus and Remus both get a chuckle out of that one. Remus then pushes a blue button and the ship takes off. Romulus is very hungry and can think of nothing else. Remus, on the other hand, can only think of the sensitive loving child he met today, Debbie.

THE END?

The creature looked up from his seat on the rock and exclaimed, "I am!"

The other creature sitting next to him said, "What do you mean, you are!"

"I mean that I am what I am and I am happy with what I am."

"This is a ridiculous conversation. Let's go on to something else. What do you want to talk about?"

"I don't know. What do you want to talk about?"

"Let's talk about the overpopulation in the cyclone area."

"No, I don't want to talk about that. Let's talk about love."

"Okay, what about it?"

"Is it okay if I ask you a question?"

"Sure, shoot!"

"What is love?"

"That is very difficult question, one that takes a lot of thought. Do you love your wife?"

"Yes, but I still don't know what it is."

"What makes you love your wife?"

"The way she treats me and takes care of me and loves me."

"So in other words, you love your wife because she loves you."

"No, I don't think so."

"Then, why do you love your wife?"

"Because I started a long time ago when we first met and now it's just a natural thing."

"There you just defined it. It's a natural thing."

"Thank-you, Hekyl."

"Your welcome, Jekyl."

THE POOR FISHERMAN

The die is cast.
The bait is attached.
All I have to do is wait,
Wait for the fish to attract.
I wonder what the fish is thinking.
I wonder if he knows the truth,
That if he comes with me he will die,
But his life will not be lost.
In death he could be admired more than in life.
He could sustain the life of another,
Thus creating the balance of nature.
The balance needed for man to survive.
And if the fish chooses to be free,
He can live as he was,
But, the poor fisherman, myself,
Will leave the pond alone,
Without the help of that fish on the line,
My time will have been for nought,
But, there is one consolation involved.
I can always come back another day and try again.

NO MATTER THE DEEDS THAT WE HAVE DONE,
THE CONCLUSION WILL COME WITH THE MORNING SUN.
WHEN THE GREAT RED BALL ARISES EVERY DAY,
THE ONLY THING TO DO IS WHAT YOU SAY.
IF YOU SPEAK WITHOUT A THOUGHT OF ACTION,
THE WORDS YOU SAY DO NOT MEAN A THING.
A THOUGHT UNSAID MIGHT AS WELL NOT HAVE BEEN THOUGHT,
BECAUSE WITHOUT AN ACTION YOU CAN NEVER GET CAUGHT.
TELLING THE TRUTH AND WITHHOLDING NOTHING IS THE KEY,
TO WHAT WE ARE AND WHAT WE MUST BE.

Bi - Pol*aroïd*

I dial the phone, but it won't ring.
You see, somebody got there before me.
I try it again, I get the same thing.
Why can't they talk after me.
I'm going to try it again right now,
so don't go away.

NEVER ENOUGH

I've seen a lot in my life,
And then again, I haven't seen enough.
I've had what one would call a wife,
But that is over with the sound of drums and a fyfe.
I've been in a place where you shouldn't be,
And I've met people there I've wished I'd never seen.
I've seen the summer color of the trees,
Turn to rainbow colors and then run free.
I've seen people dying and I've seen people crying.
I've seen people living and I've seen people laughing.
I've seen it all, yet, I haven't seen enough.

Oct. 5, 1978
I am 24.

What is life without love?
What is love without life?
They are equally distressing and depressing.

Life without love = Dead subject

BRUCE'S SURPRISE BIRTHDAY PARTY

'TIS THAT TIME OF YEAR AGAIN.
EVERYBODY HAS ONE; BUT WHY THIS?
ON MY BIRTHDAY, I DON'T EVEN GET CARDS.
NOW THERE'S BRUCE'S SURPRISE BIRTHDAY PARTY.
I WONDER TO MYSELF SOMETIMES,
WOULDN'T IT BE NEAT IF SOMEONE DID THAT FOR ME.
WHAT A FANTASTIC FEELING OF
ONENESS WITH MANKIND.
BUT, ALAS IT SHALL NEVER HAPPEN TO ME.
I'VE NOT BEEN ABLE TO FIND SOMEONE
AS SPECIAL AS DEBBIE!
P.S. WELCOME BACK FITZ!

LOVERS AND OTHER STRANGERS/DEBBIE

SHE'S BEAUTIFUL AND ALL THE
THINGS I FIND APPEALING,
AND I KEEP THINKING TO MYSELF,
WHY CAN'T I HAVE HER?
THE ANSWER IS CLEAR; SHE TOLD ME HERSELF,
EITHER WE ARE FRIENDS AND NOT LOVERS
OR LOVERS AND NOT FRIENDS.
SO, UNFORTUNATELY, THAT IS WHERE
OUR FURTHER RELATIONSHIP ENDS.
BUT FRIENDS WE ARE AND THE BEST OF FRIENDS, TOO,
AND THANK GOD IN THIS CASE
THERE IS NO PAYMENT DUE.
SHE IS A REAL PERSON THAT HELPS
BEFORE SHE KNOWS WHY.
SHE ALLOWED ME TO MATURE INTO THE PERSON
THAT I HAVE ALWAYS WANTED TO BE.
AND GIVEN ME THE STRENGTH TO CARRY
ON WHEN THINGS WERE TOUGH.
TO SAY I LOVE THIS PERSON WOULD
ONLY TEND TO SADDEN ME,
SINCE FRIENDS CAN NEVER BE LOVERS.

REFRAIN
LOVERS AND OTHER STRANGERS
WHAT COULD BE THE DANGERS.
AND, A FOOL IS ONE WHO ANGERS,
OVER LOVERS AND OTHER STRANGERS.

Chapter 3

Second Chance

"Hey, let me out of here. I don't like being fenced up like this."

Nobody hears him or they pretend not to hear him.

He tries again. "If you don't let me out of here, I'm going to tell my friend Iggy on all of you."

Still, there is silence from the people around him.

He thinks for a moment. Where am I anyway? Then, suddenly, the aroma reaches him. Even though he is trapped and he can't move, he can still smell. "That sure smells good," he thinks out loud.

Just then, he hears a voice. "I sure am hungry, Mommy. I can't wait any longer! What time are we going to eat?"

"As soon as your daddy gets home from work, Jesse," says his mother.

The voices stop.

I'm starting to get scared, he says to himself. What am I going to do?

He hears a voice again. "Jesse, I'm going out back to water the flowers. Please try to stay out of trouble, okay?"

"Yes, Mommy," replies Jesse.

The voices stop, again, but he hears a creaking sound. He hears a voice from far away. "Jesse, remind me to tell your father to oil this door!"

Then he is alone with this boy, Jesse. I can't see in here, he thinks. Then the idea hits him. Maybe if I yell for help very loudly, this boy will be able to hear me!

"Help me, help me, I'm trapped in here, help!!!" he screams.

Jesse turns and stares at the kitchen counter. I thought I heard something, he thinks. I guess not.

But, the voice comes again. "Please help me," he screams even louder, "please, I need help!"

This time Jesse knows he hears something. It sounds to him like a whisper. He walks over to the kitchen counter and looks at the food his mother has been preparing for dinner.

"Rescue me, please, I need your help!"

Jesse knows where the sound is coming from now. What do I do? he thinks. Who ever heard of a whispering corndog? He picks up the corndog and turns it to see what could possibly be making that noise.

"Please, put me down. I am afraid of heights!" squeals the corndog, scared yet relieved to be rescued.

Jesse puts the corndog down, quickly, but gently. He stands thinking for a second, then speaks.

"How do you talk like that?"

No answer.

Jesse scratches his head and then decides to inspect this mysterious corndog. At first look, he doesn't see or hear a thing. After a while, though, he hears the whispering again. He puts his ear to the corndog and listens. He hears his dinner say, "Let me out of here, it's getting hard to breathe!"

Jesse knows immediately what he has to do. He puts his hand on the stick and with the other hand, he starts to push up the corn meal jacket the hotdog is wearing. It pushes up easily enough. Pretty soon, all the covering is removed from the hotdog. He sees absolutely nothing strange about the hotdog! He hears the voice again, though. It is still muffled so he puts his ear close to the hotdog again and this is what the little boy hears, "Turn me over, turn me over!"

Fear hits Jesse all of a sudden, but curiousity has been working on him for such a long time. I have to turn it over, he thinks. So, he does.

"Hey, what are you staring at?" says the hotdog. "Haven't you ever seen a pig before?"

Jesse replies. "You're not a pig. You're a hotdog."

"Can't you see, I'm a pig?!"

"No, you're not a pig. You're a hotdog, but you sure are strange. You have two brown eyes looking up at me, a hole for a nose and a big hole for your mouth."

The mystery is starting to unravel for the hotdog. The last he remembers, he was on a truck with all of his friends and they were let off next to some big building. Now I remember, he thinks, there were men killing all my friends and I was next!! I'm dead!!! No, I'm not, I'm a hotdog now. Someone has given me one more chance on a stick.

"Don't eat me," cries the hotdog. "I'm still alive!"

Jesse can't understand what is going on. He is only seven, but he knows one thing. He is not going to eat *that* hotdog!

"Okay," says Jesse, "I won't eat you, but what are we going to do? My mother is going to come back in here any minute."

Just then, the hotdog hears a familiar sound. It's a dog, says the hotdog, this time to himself. The barking comes closer and closer.

Jesse speaks, "Get away from there, CoCo. Go sit in the corner!"

The dog doesn't listen, of course. They never listen to kids.

Jesse hears the creaking of the back door. Quickly, he hides the hotdog in the breadbox and walks swiftly over to the kitchen sink. His mother enters the room. She looks at CoCo barking at the kitchen counter, then at Jesse standing innocently in front of the sink and finally at the kitchen counter. She says, "What is going on in here, Jesse? What is that damn dog barking at?"

"I don't know," says Jesse, trying to smile.

"CoCo, go sit in the corner, now!" yells Jesse's mother.

CoCo puts her tail between her legs and walks slowly over to the corner. She sits in the corner, but her eyes are still staring at the kitchen counter.

"Jesse, I want to know what is going on here," says his mother, trying to sound calm. She always has better luck with Jesse when he thinks his mother isn't mad at him.

"Mommy, you're not going to believe what I have to say."

"Try me."

"Alright," says Jesse, trying to stall it off for as long as he can. When he sees his mother's eyes start to widen, he decides it is time to talk. Then, quickly, he says, "There is a talking hotdog in the breadbox."

"What?" says his mother.

"I heard the corndog whispering so I peeled off the corn meal and there was this talking hotdog. If you don't believe me, look for yourself."

Jesse's mother's name is Sandy. She has been married to Sam Golden for the last ten years. During the past five years, she has seen her son, Jesse, tell a lot of tall tales, but this one is too much. She doesn't know what to say or what to do.

"Hey, let me out of here. I can't stand being fenced up anymore," screams the hotdog from the breadbox.

Sandy can not believe her ears. CoCo begins to bark in the corner. Jesse runs over to the breadbox and takes his hotdog out of its prison.

"Thanks, Jesse," says the hotdog "You saved my life, again."

Sandy's mouth has dropped until it is almost touching the floor. CoCo has run over to Jesse and is barking up at the hotdog in his hand.

Suddenly, Jesse's mind starts to race. He hears his father's car door slam and he knows his father is home. Jesse's father is almost never in a good mood when he comes home from work. He is a meat packer which scares him even more now that he has a hotdog in his hand that he wants to keep alive.

This whole time, the hotdog has been screaming about his fear of heights and the dog barking up at him. He begins to feel faint. Jesse hears the cries, finally, and puts the hotdog down on the kitchen counter just as his father opens the front door.

"What's happening here!" exclaims Sam Golden.

The only answer he gets is silence. Even the hotdog is quiet now. Jesse glances over at the kitchen counter and notices that the face on his hotdog has vanished. His mother's voice interrupts his thoughts.

"Nothing is going on, darling. We just needed you to come home now."

"Oh," says Sam, "what's for supper?"

"We are having steak and Jesse is having a cor . . ., I mean, hotdog."

Jesse speaks. "Hi, Dad." He is surprised at how controlled his voice is. He continues. "I'm not very hungry tonight. I've got a stomach ache. Can I be excused from dinner?"

"Sure, son, but you go lay down if you're not feeling well."

"Okay, Daddy."

Jesse starts to walk away from his parents toward the stairs to his bedroom. He overhears his father saying to his mother, "You don't look so well either, Sandy. You look like you've just seen a ghost." As he goes up the stairs, the sound of his parents' voices fade away.

He starts to think about the hotdog. It must have died, he says to himself. I will never eat another hotdog *ever* again.

He quickly runs up the rest of the stairs to his bedroom and then takes a flying leap onto his bed. Jesse lays back and while thinking about the hotdog, hears his stomach rumbling. He remembers his hunger and his mind begins to wander. He pictures in his thoughts the nice juicy steak he knows his Dad is eating right now. He cannot stop his mouth from watering.

Falling

Alfred fell and he couldn't stop falling and then suddenly he woke up. The sweat was laden all over his body. He felt weak and drained, yet curious. I was dreaming. he thought, and I was dreaming about falling, but I can't remember what I was dreaming about.

Alfred decided to get up and get a drink of something cold to make himself feel better. He was startled by the cold rush of air as he opened the refrigerator door. He took out the bottle of apple juice, took a drink, and replaced it in the refrigerator.

He looked at his watch. It was 2:30 A.M. I'm not really tired, he thought, but maybe I should try and get some sleep.

Just then, there was a knock on the door, He looked at the door, looked again at his watch, then back at the door. Who could it be at this hour?

"Who is it?" Alfred said, trying to hide his fear.

No answer.

Well, it must have been my imagination, he thought, and he decided to go back to sleep. As he approached his bedroom door, he heard the knocking again, this time louder than before. He jumped and looked at the front door. The knocking came again!

"Who is it?" Alfred said, this time not being able to hold back the fear.

Still no answer.

He pinched himself to see if he was awake; he was. Then, he remembered the peep-hole in his door. He walked slowly over to the door and looked out the peep-hole. He didn't see a thing.

A voice from the other side spoke, "Let me in, I'm shot!" The voice sounded weak and hurt.

Alfred stood and thought for a minute. Should I open the door and possibly involve myself in something? I can't just leave him out there bleeding. Or, is he really hurt?

For some reason, Alfred felt compelled to open the door. What he saw on the other side of the door took his breath away. The man was not lying, he was shot in the leg, but the kind of man he was took Alfred aback. His face was a greenish color, he was short and he looked very alien.

Alfred hesitated, but he asked a question, "Who are *you*?!"

"I am Lucas from the planet, Aquarius. Help me get back to my spaceship. I will be alright if I can just get back to my ship."

"Alright, "said Alfred, "let me get into some clothes."

Alfred returned shortly, dressed looking a whiter shade of pale, but ready to do what he felt he must. He picked up the green man and started to walk.

"Where is your ship?" asked Alfred.

"Just over the hill."

Alfred walked for a long time, but Lucas was not very heavy, so the trip was not all that difficult. Lucas felt strange to the touch, something that really gave Alfred the chills, but he figured, the faster I walk, the sooner I can get this over with.

Soon, they reached the spaceship. The door opened automatically and Lucas motioned Alfred to step on board the ship. No sooner had he stepped foot inside the spaceship, then the door closed and the spaceship took off.

"Let me out of here!!" Alfred cried.

"Okay, "said Lucas, "but you humans sure are strange!"

The door of the spaceship opened and Lucas pushed Alfred out. Alfred fell, and he couldn't stop falling and then suddenly he remembered what he was dreaming about.

THE END

Part II

The sky was black and there was not a cloud in the sky. Out of it came a sudden burst of flames like that of a back fire on a car. The spaceship hovered over the village, waiting for the right time; the right time to land.

"Hey, Romulus," asks Remus, "how does this place fit in with the rest of our plans?"

"Well you see, Remus," answers Romulus, "our mission is to explore other planets and seek out new ideas. I think we can learn something from this place."

"Okay, then let's land already. I'm getting hungry."

The ship hesitates for just a moment, then lands in the middle of a valley. The door of the spaceship opens to reveal two very small green men slowly emerging from the interior of their slim-lined Model A.

"Where are we anyway?" asks Remus.

"We are back on the asteroid of Capernicus, Remus. Don't you remember going for the gold?"

"Oh, yeh," laughs Remus, "but why are we back again?"

Romulus thinks for just a short while, then he begins to walk away from the ship. Remus follows him quickly and they climb up a hill to a wooden structure built about the size of these two creatures from the sky. Romulus opens the gate and promptly steps through the door.

A look of disgust appears on his face. Then, suddenly Remus smells it, too. Romulus has just stepped in god shit.

Romulus speaks. "Please, Remus, go back to the ship and get me a tissue for my feet!"

"Yes, sir!" and Remus is gone in a flash!

Part III

"Splat!"
"Splat!"
"That's it!" exclaims Remus with a huge amount of glee.
Romulus, who has found that you need more than a tissue to remove god shit, answers Remus in a tone reserved for very sad ocassions. "What is it, Remus?"
"I have figured out how god shit sounds; the sound that has been heard throughout human's existence. The sound is:"
Romulus has walked away from Remus and is starting to investigate the human abode in front him. Remus, meanwhile, has paused for extreme dramatic effect.
"Splat!!!"

Ted Berkowitz stared at the sky, but he just couldn't believe what he saw. About a meter above his head hovered what appeared to be a space vehicle. He could feel his stomach tightening as fear began rushing through his veins.

The United States had space vehicles like that, but not ships that looked as strange! It was shaped like a ball and had a trail of smoke from its disappearing end.

Now it was coming back at him. It must have seen me, he thought. In that instant he began running as fast as he could toward his house. He looked over his shoulder to see if it was following him and it was!

The knot in his stomach had grown to an enormous size by then and he thought for sure that it was going to burst. His legs kept on churning, though his mind was in the throes of agony.

What was this thing?

What did it want with him?

Why was it chasing him?

These were all questions which his mind could not answer.

ROMULUS & REMUS PART IV

"ROMULUS, WHY WON'T YOU TELL ME WHY WE ARE HERE."

"WE ARE HERE TO VISIT DAVID. HE WAS THE GUY WITH DEBBIE WHEN WE WENT FOR THE GOLD IN 1979. NOW HE'S GOT A WIFE AND HER NAME IS TERRIE. SHE'S SUPPOSED TO BE A HOT DISH," EXCLAIMS REMUS WITH GLEE!

REMUS SCRATCHES HIS HEAD, THEN DECIDES TO STEP OUTSIDE TO ACTIVATE THE CLOAKING DEVICE ON THE SPACE SHIP. ON THE WAY BACK, HE REALIZES THAT THE NAME OF DAVID SAMUELSON IS A NAME HE HAS HEARD BEFORE.

ROMULUS WAITS PATIENTLY FOR THE ARRIVAL OF HIS LONG TIME FRIEND REMUS. REMUS FELL IN LOVE WITH DEBBIE THE LAST TIME WE WERE HERE.

REMUS ARRIVED BACK AND LOOKED IN WONDER AT THE ARCHITECTURE THAT WAS SURROUNDING HIM. AND THEN, SUDDENLY, HE THOUGHT OF DEBBIE AND ALL THAT CAME INTO HIS HEAD IS THE ASSHOLE THAT TOOK HER AWAY, BRUCE.

REMUS DECIDES THAT DAYDREAMING IS FOR THE SDRIB. COMING TO HIS MIND INSTEAD IS DAVID, THE MANIC-DEPRESSIVE.

REMUS THINKS VERY HARD INTO THE BACK OF HIS TINY BRAIN AND SEES THE OTHER HOSPITALIZATIONS.

ROMULUS STARTS WALKING BACK TOWARDS THE OLD MODEL A, THE MOST DEPENDABLE SHIP IN THE GALAXY. "REMUS, COME ON, WE HAVE TO GO. I'M GETTING VERY HUNGRY!"

"OKAY, BUT I'M JUST SORRY THAT WE'VE NEVER MET DAVID SAMUELSON FACE TO FACE. ALAS AND WOE IS ME."

THE TWO FRIENDS CLIMB ABOARD THEIR SHIP AND INSTANTLY TAKE OFF FOR WORLDS UNKNOWN.

HI, I'M DAVID SAMUELSON AND I HOPE YOU HAVE ENJOYED MY WRITING. I WISH, TO ALL MANKIND, A HOPE THAT PARENTS DON'T DO WHAT MY PARENTS DID TO ME. THEY STIFLED ME AND DID NOT ALLOW ME TO GAIN MY OWN IDENTITY OR EVEN DEVELOP FEELINGS. FEELINGS OF LOVE, HATE AND SO MANY MORE. I DON'T LIVE THAT WAY NOW. I HAVE THREE CHILDREN, TWO STEPCHILDREN WHOM I LOVE AND ONE SON. IF THIS IS A HAPPY ENDING TO THIS BOOK, THEN I HAD BETTER STOP. GOOD LUCK TO YOU AND REMEMBER TO THINK SAFETY!

ROMULUS AND REMUS HAD JUST TOUCHED DOWN IN HEDRON. THE ANTICIPATION OF A GOOD TIME WAS EVIDENT.

"HEY ROMULUS," SAYS REMUS EXCITEDLY. "HOW COME THE TEMPERATURE IS SO LOW HERE? THE TEMPERATURE IS SUPPOSED TO BE NEAR ONE HUNDRED. THE TEMPERATURE IS ONLY EIGHTY-SEVEN."

"VERY INTERESTING, REMUS. BUT, YOU KNOW THE ANSWER TO THAT! THE COLD FRONT CAME THROUGH THIRTEEN HOURS AGO AND THAT IS THE DIFFERENCE IN THE TEMPERATURE."

"OH." REMUS PAUSES FOR JUST A SECOND AND SAYS, "YOU DON'T EXPECT ME TO BELIEVE THAT BULLSHIT, DO YOU?"

"JUST TESTING, REMUS, JUST TESTING."

NOW IS THE TIME FOR ALL GOOD MEN
TO COME TO THE AID OF THEIR WOMEN.
YOU SEE, IT IS NOW THAT WE HAVE COME,
TO THE YEAR OF ROMULUS & REMUS.

"HEY, ROMULUS," CALLS REMUS VERY EXCITEDLY. "WHAT'S THAT?"

ROMULUS LOOKS AT THE VIEWING SCREEN ON THE SHELF IN THEIR SPACE SHIP AT WHICH REMUS IS POINTING AT. ROMULUS SPEAKS. "THAT MY DEAR REMUS, IS A GAME CALLED "FOOTBALL"."

"THAT'S NO GAME, ROMULUS. LOOK AT THE WAY THOSE CAPERNICUS MEN ARE HITTING EACH OTHER. THAT'S NO GAME. THAT'S A WAR!"

"NOW, REMUS, DON'T GET LIKE THAT. IT IS A GAME OF WIN OR LOSE, AND NEITHER TEAM WANTS TO BE THE LOSER."

"EXPLAIN SOMETHING ELSE TO ME, ROMULUS. WHAT PART DOES THE "REFRIGERATOR" PLAY IN THIS GAME CALLED FOOTBALL?"

ROMULUS FEELS A JOKE COMING ON. HIS SIDES START TO LAUGH, BUT THE REST OF HIM STAYS CALM. REMUS STARES AT ROMULUS IN WONDERMENT. HE DOESN'T HAVE A CHANCE TO SEE ROMULUS ENJOYING HIMSELF VERY MUCH.

"REMUS, THE REFRIGERATOR'S PURPOSE IS TO COOL OFF THE OTHER TEAM."

REMUS CAN'T BELIEVE IT, BUT ROMULUS HAS TOLD A BAD JOKE! "THAT'S FUNNY, ROMULUS, BUT WHAT ABOUT THIS ONE. WHY DID THE REFRIGERATOR CROSS THE ROAD?"

ROMULUS ACTUALLY BEGINS TO LAUGH WATCHING THE BIG MEN RUN AND JUMP AND KNOCK HEADS WITH THEIR TEAMMATES. "THE ANSWER TO YOUR QUESTION REMUS IS; TO GET TO THE OTHER SIDE."

"FUNNY, ROMULUS. BUT THE REAL ANSWER IS: TO CHASE HIS "GOD"!"

I AM MANIC RIGHT NOW, AND I CAN FEEL IT IN MY HEAD. IT FEELS HOT AND WARM, FULL OF THOUGHTS AND

ACTIONS; AND IT CAN'T STOP. MARIJUANA STIMULATES ME LIKE THIS AND WILL WEAR OFF ALL TOO SOON. IN THE MEANTIME, HERE'S ROMULUS AND REMUS.

ROMULUS AND REMUS AGAIN FIND THEMSELVES CIRCLING THE ASTEROID, CAPERNICUS. HUNGER IS A REAL NEED FOR THEM AS ALWAYS.

"HEY, ROMULUS, LET'S GO DOWN THERE AND GET SOME GOOD "ACAB" MEAT. MAYBE WE COULD EVEN EAT "ATAXI" THIS TIME." REMUS CAN'T HELP BUT CHUCKLE AT HIS OWN JOKE.

ROMULUS REPLIES. "REMUS, MY MISGUIDED FRIEND, YOU ARE SO SELFISH SOMETIMES. YOU *KNOW* WHAT WE HAVE TO DO DOWN THERE. THIS IS SERIOUS BUSINESS!"

"OH, GEE ROMULUS. SOMETIMES I GET SO HUNGRY I COULD EAT AN "ESROH"." REMUS CLEARS HIS THROAT AND THEN FINALLY REALIZING WHAT THEY WERE GOING TO DO, CHOKES BACK A TEAR. "ALRIGHT," REMUS BLURTS OUT, "LET'S GET IT OVER WITH!"

ROMULUS AND REMUS ARRIVE AT THE WALKER PLACE VERY EARLY IN THE MORNING. THE PLACE IS DARK AND THE "GOD" AND THE REST OF THE FAMILY ARE ASLEEP.

"I BET THEY DON'T WANT TO LOSE IT," SAYS REMUS SADLY.

"THERE IS AN EVENTUALITY IN THESE "ACAB'S" LIVES, DEATH. AND BESIDES THAT, REMUS, IT REMAINS SURVIVAL OF THE FITTEST."

THEY SLIP THROUGH THE OUTSIDE OF THE HOUSE AND HEAD FOR THE STAIRS. SOON THEY ARE UPSTAIRS WHERE DAVID AND TERRIE SLEEP. THEY SEE THE "GOD" SLEEPING ON A BLANKET IN THE CORNER OF THE ROOM. REMUS GLANCES AT THE TWO SLEEPING "ACABS" IN THE ROOM.

"I CAN'T STAND IT, ROMULUS! I CAN'T STAND A "REDNER REDRUM"!"

"I KNOW, REMUS, BUT WE NEED TO TAKE IT OUT OF ITS MISERY. YOU CAN'T BACK OUT ON ME. WE HAVE TO DO THIS. A "GOD" IS TO BE RESPECTED, AND WE MUST GRANT HER THIS LAST FINAL WISH."

THEY PICK UP THE "GOD" GENTLY AND TAKE IT DOWN THE STAIRS. THE "GOD" SLIPS THROUGH THE WALLS LIKE ROMULUS AND REMUS DO, BUT STILL CONTINUES TO SLEEP.

"WHERE CAN WE FIND A "DUTS" THIS TIME OF THE MORNING?" ASKS REMUS WITH A STOPPING START.

"DON'T WORRY. I HAVE THE PLAN THOUGHT OUT TO THE LAST FINAL DETAIL," REPLIES ROMULUS.

THE "GOD" WAKES UP FINALLY AND SEES HER FINAL WISH IN FRONT OF HER EYES. SHE APPROACHES HER "DUTS" WITH GREAT TREPIDATION. YOU SEE, SHE'S NEVER DONE IT BEFORE.

"HEY ROMULUS! YOU THINK THAT "GOD" IS GOING TO LET THAT "DUTS" AT HER?"

"OF COURSE!" REPLIES ROMULUS WITH CERTAINTY. "THESE "ACABS" MUST ALWAYS HAVE A NEW AND DIFFERENT "GOD". THEY WILL PERFORM THE ACT, REMUS. YOU WILL SEE."

SOON ENOUGH, ROMULUS WAS PROVEN RIGHT. THE "GOD" HAD SEEN HER LAST FEW MINUTES OF GLORY WITH THE GREATEST OF PLEASURE. ROMULUS AND REMUS HEAD BACK FOR THEIR SHIP, ANOTHER "REDNER REDRUM" COMPLETE.

"YOU KNOW WHAT WE FORGOT, REMUS? WE FORGOT TO GET SOMETHING TO EAT!"

"HOW CAN YOU THINK OF EATING AT A TIME LIKE THIS?" REMUS PAUSES FOR A MOMENT, THEN SAYS VERY SLOWLY, "LET'S GIVE THE "GOD" A FEW MINUTES OF SILENT PRAYER BEFORE WE EAT."

A FEW MINUTES LATER, THE "REDNER REDRUM" FORGOTTEN, THEY EAT SOME FRESH "REGRUB" LIKE THE ANIMALS THEY REALLY ARE!

1979

At times like this I sit and think,
Of all the things that I have.
And when I think of my love Terrie,
My heart begins to sing.

Robin and Mindy are more for me,
Then I could ever ask for.
They are warm and sweet and lovable.
And I love them more and, more.

There's an awful lot that I have right now,
With soon a wife and two children.
It excites me and makes me happy,
Happier than I have ever been

Chapter 4

(Eighteen and over only - X rated)

$E = mc^2$

Erection = marrying with two children or mother and two children

MY LOVE

How can I tell you how I feel?
All I have are words.
And words are no guarantee or salvation,
But, that is all I have.
You see, your beauty warms me inside.
It makes me want to hold you, to touch you, to feel you.
It eminates from every part of you,
Sometimes more inside, sometimes more outwardly,
But it is always present.
Your goodness shows everytime you smile.
You want someone else to feel good. G-d what a quality!
This poem could go on forever,
You see, I love you, Terrie,
But, words are cheap these days.
Just one more thing, though.
My love for you will never die,
It will go on and on and on.

FORTIFICATION FOR THE CAR WHILE DEPRESSED IN MID '80'S

SO, I'M DEPRESSED! I CAN STILL FUNCTION AND MY I.Q. IS THE SAME AS ALWAYS. JUST WHEN THINGS GET THE WORST, IT GETS BETTER. SELF-CONFIDENCE IS MISSING, BUT YOU CAN STILL FLY.

WELL, THERE'S NOTHING WORSE THAN A PASSING FRIEND,
WHO WILL DIE ON YOU TILL THE BITTER END.
THERE'S NOTHING WORSE THAN A BURNING HEART,
OR A PAST THAT TEARS THE WORLD APART.
                    BOY GEORGE

DO YOU REALLY WANT TO HURT ME?
DO YOU REALLY WANT TO MAKE ME CRY?
DO YOU REALLY WANT TO HURT ME?
DO YOU REALLY WANT TO MAKE ME CRY!
                    BOY GEORGE

LAID BACK UPTOWN TURNAROUND PEOPLE
WEAR DISGUISES.
THEY LIE, SO SORRY IS THE WORD
THAT'S ALL THEY EVER NEED
TO FORGIVE MY YESTERDAYS.
SORRY BY RAY THOMAS

Dec. 14, 1985

Lake Worth, Florida

They fall asleep together.
They wake up apart.
But, no one can tell whether,
Six years is a big head start.
Seven years is too big a head start.
He did time for being very bad,
She had little time for being sad,
They grew up so very differently.
But, their love is all that you can see.

SHE IS LOVELY YET RESERVED.
HER VOICE WILL SOON BE HEARD,
WHILE WE THINK AND PRAY
FOR THOSE THAT CANNOT ON THIS DAY.

SHE IS POLITE YET SHY.
HER VOICE WILL SOON BE HEARD,
ON THIS DAY OF HER THIRTEENTH YEAR
WHICH MEANS SO MUCH TO HER AND THOSE DEAR.

SHE IS VERY INTENT AND VERY KIND,
AND HER VOICE YOU WILL SURELY FIND,
WILL HELP US TO UNITE TOGETHER
FOR A JOYOUS AND MEMORABLE DAY.

                          Robin's Bat Mitzvah

In a town called Walnut Grove, lives a family called the Ingalls. In the Ingalls family there are four girls, Mary, Laura, Carrie and Grace. They have a Ma named Caroline and a Pa named Charles. The year is 1874. During the day, Pa works as a carpenter. Ma stays home with Carrie who is three and Grace who is one. Laura and Mary go to school in town.

Today is a beautiful spring day; a day to go to the fair. Charles, Caroline, and Mary decide that Mary has a say in what she thinks is the best because she is 15.

When they get there, the heat meets them first. The day is much hotter than expected. Laura wants to go and see the pigs first. She likes to watch them play in the mud.

Mary, on the other hand, is helping Carrie on one of the rides. Carrie wants to go on the pony ride, so Mary volunteers.

Ma and Pa decide to look at all the many things they can buy at the fair. There are many fancy belt buckles, shirts and dresses. Anything a body could ever want.

Then suddenly, the wind starts to blow like the thunder. The rain starts to fall all around the Ingalls family. The first thing that happens is, Carrie falls off her pony. Then, Laura falls in to the pig pen. Mary holds on to a pole, which holds her up very well. Ma and Pa are having a heck of a time trying to stand on their own two feet

As suddenly as it had come, the storm flies away. Carrie, whose arm, really hurts her, runs crying to Ma and Pa still brushing the mud off of their clothes. Laura has made friends with one of the pigs. Mary, on the other hand, is walking blindly and weakly over to where her family is standing.

The wind blows strongly again on our fearless friends. The rain keeps falling and keeps on falling until the water is up to Pa's waist. Luckily, he carries Carrie on his shoulders or she surely would have drowned. Laura is on top of the pig pen holding tightly onto her friend Iggy. But, nobody knows where Mary is.

When the storm finally clears the air is calm and the sky is bright and blue. Ma, Pa, Laura, Carrie and Iggy stand in the center of where once stood a very fine fair. You see, if it wasn't for their good friend Iggy, they never would have made it. Laura, who is already standing on the pig pen, yells over to Ma and Pa, "Swim over here to me!"

Pa says, "I can't. I've got Carrie on my head. I can't swim with Carrie on my head!"

Ma speaks for the first time. "Charles, why don't we just walk through the water. It's not over our heads."

"Good idea, Ma," cries Pa.

They start to walk very slowly through the high waters to their favorite daughter. When they get there, Laura takes Carrie off of Pa's head. Pa and Ma then climb up onto the pig pen and everybody is miraculously saved from the terrible storm.

As I said, the storm has broken now. Everybody is talking about just how hungry they are. Crying, Carrie says, "I'm hungry! Where's Mary?," over and over again.

JAN. 27, 1986
1:30 A.M.

The Chicago Bears just won the Super Bowl. Isn't that amazing? My parents are in Phoenix and the pay off for Dakota Packing is just four days away. The general ledger goes on my computer system today. Also, today is the day that I begin to buy a new house on Dunham Place. I can't believe this is all happening to me. It's too good to be true. This is what you might call: a Chicago success story.

Headlines: Manic-Depressive makes it big in Chicago.

FEBRUARY 15, 1986

DEAR DIARY:
I HAVE WORKED FOR A LONG TIME TO GET TO THIS POINT AND NO ONE IS GOING TO TAKE IT AWAY FROM ME.

It's finally over! The hurricane seems to be over! It's time to see (The Sting) and buy a new house. Out of the blue, my new red GL Subaru will be ready Wednesday or Thursday. I will see Chuck and Debbie tonight. I hope they don't smoke too much.

Secret Messages!

I told John today that the thing to do right now is to lease a car. It cost $150.00 a month to lease a nice car.

I need to call Aurelio Rodriguez to see if any of his friends might like to buy a great townhouse.

Hold on Tight to Your Dream

Jeff Lynne

Why can't a Jewish lady get a colostomy?

Because she can't find shoes to match the bag!

Chapter 5

(Eighteen and over only - X rated)

Seven years is a bigger head start,
And if we are not going to fall apart,
We better get going, and into bed,
So that you can give me the greatest head!

May 18, 1986

Four weeks of unemployment,
Sobers a man to the fact,
That jobs are not heaven sent,
Nor the pain and stress compact.

But, with helping friends like you,
I found a job in just three weeks.
Still, I am sure you'd say this too,
"Unemployment really reeks!"

David Samuelson
Hallmark Pool Corporation
2785 Algonquin Road
Rolling Meadows, IL 60008

MINDY'S BAT MITZVAH

I'VE WATCHED YOU GROW,
FROM BABY CRIB UNTIL THIS DAY;
BODY IN MOTION, CONSTANTLY ON THE GO,
WITH KIND THINGS TO SAY TO ALL WE KNOW.

MAY THIS DAY BRING YOU AS MUCH JOY,
AS YOU HAVE BROUGHT TO MY LIFE,
AND MAY THERE BE VERY LITTLE STRIFE,
IN THE DAYS OF THE REST OF YOUR LIFE.

2/14/91

This being our *thirteenth* Valentine's Day,
It's special to me in more than one way,
The love we have shared for all these years,
Makes life worth living; through all our fears.
And, on this lucky day, I love you, Terrie,
With hopes and wishes, we will always make merry!

Chapter 6

My World of Work - Post Pop-In - Renaissance Man

Authority. My father was my boss for many years. I was afraid of my father. A little history: My father and mother came to this country in the late thirties chased by Hitler and his hired henchmen. My father became a butcher and worked his way into a corporate partnership in a wholesale meat packing company called Dakota Packing Co. My father, at home, when I was young, was distant, constantly sleeping, angry and a great fear in my life. Later, when I started working for him, getting up at 4:00 A.M., getting home at between 6:00 P.M. and 9:00 P.M., I saw a much different side of my father I never saw before. He was happy, constantly swearing, a leader, extroverted to a degree and confident. Quite a change for me to see. Enough history.

A lot of the communication I had with my father's partners, I believe, was tempered by the fact that I was their partner's son. Here is an example of an interaction with my father. At one point during my promotions within Dakota Packing, along with my salary raise, I had requested three weeks vacation because I had just gotten married and my wife liked to spend a couple of weeks with her family on the east coast. Whenever I asked for something from my father, I tried to make sure the request would be understood by him and that I would have little chance of being rejected. In this case, my father said okay and that was that. Or so I thought. Maybe a month later my father approached me saying I have to give back what he said about the three weeks vacation. It seemed that Roger, the general manager, only had two weeks vacation and they didn't want Roger to be hurt. I disagreed with him, but not too forcefully. But, I was very upset. I'm sure it affected my work, my sleep and my family life greatly. When something hits me like that, I get very upset. I talked to my wife on the phone from work constantly about it and I'm sure my attitude toward the company changed during

89

that time. I finally decided to talk to my father about it again. (I waited until I was calm and rational.) I told him that I thought his decision was completely unfair and that he should talk to his partners about giving Roger three weeks vacation. In retrospect, the fear of losing my job was ever prevalent, (the ultimate rejection), but I didn't believe that my father would fire me. I guess I felt I had something on him because I was his son.

When I went to Hallmark Pool Corp., Kim and Jack, my bosses, during my offer of a job, told me that a stock portion of the company would be in my future if things went well in our relationship. How did this affect me? It made me work like the dickens. You see working for my father was like working for my own business and I worked as if that was true. Working for my father gave me a feeling of security and, for the most part, I was happy working there. This left me a bit naive when it came to being manipulated by my boss. For example, Kim always told me when I was leaving for the day at an hour earlier then he wanted me to go, sarcastically, "Leaving early today, huh?" He would still be there and would be at all odd hours waiting for his girlfriends to come by. At those times, I would leave, but I would feel very concerned about leaving again early because he would "criticize" me again for leaving early. By the way, "early" was getting there at 8:00 A.M. and leaving between 6:00 and 7:00 P.M. The way I got a smile or a pat on the back or decent talk was if I stayed to close to 8:00 P.M. I guess I allowed him to manipulate me, even at the expense of my family, the relationship outside activities or whatever else. During the time I spent at Hallmark Pool Corp. in which I worked my tail off, I was not happy due, I think, in part to the realization that it was not my business and not knowing what to do about it. Also, because of the manipulation. During the next two years, I was rewarded with raises, trips to both Las Vegas and Milwaukee, but no stock. Finally a confrontation with Kim on the idea revealed the fact that I was getting no stock. Even though I was unhappy most of the time, that was the beginning of the end. When U.S. Pool, a start-up company, offered me a job with a pay increase, I jumped ship.

While still at Hallmark Pool, I had the opportunity to meet with a consultant who advised me that a controller's job could and should be done in a forty-five hour week. So, going into my next two jobs, I told my bosses that I would only be working forty-five hours. They both cooperated. My relationship with the boss at U.S. Pool Corp. was short lived. We seemed to respect each other. Here's the vignette: It was toward the end of my two months there. Money was needed to continue the business. Richard offered me 5% stock if I could find money to keep it going. Again, this gave me a rush to try, but time ran out quickly. He couldn't pay me. Either he give me that 5% of stock or I was leaving. He turned me down and I left.

Bernie was my next boss. He went along with my forty-five hour request. He was also desperate since his controller wanted to leave and was having a nervous breakdown at the same time. Bernie was also very sick, rarely at work; and his wife, who was once a major part of the business, had an advanced case of Alzeimer's disease. The supermarket, solely owned by Bernie, was in the worst black neighborhood of Chicago and it was losing money like crazy. (Don't say it!) When Bernie was around or on the phone, I was afraid of him as was everybody else. That lasted a year. If you are interested in why I was afraid, I will explain it in discussion.

My last bosses, seven millionaires, made a wrong decision in aquiring Pop-In Supermarket. They never interviewed or talked to me their CEO (general manager), they just gave me the title and responsibility. First, though, they gave me the title of CEO which was quite a rush for me Of course, I found out later it was just a game to get me going. As far as communication with my bosses, it set up a situation where I had a boss one morning a week between 6:00 - 7:30 A.M. (for breakfast) and that was the extent of having a boss. They basically wanted me to run it on my own with little prior supermarket experience. My breakfast meetings with Ed went one of two ways. (Generalizing a little.) I would present situations and problems, things I had done, some financial information, advertising, etc . . . His reaction to me would be to ask me questions, like what do you think, to gain solutions to problems. Or on some occasions, he would offer his opinions, which I took, which proved to be a mistake. The other way our meetings went was for Ed to tell me, after hearing me out, that he did not want to hear problems, he wanted to hear only solutions. Either way, at the end of our breakfast, he would usually hit me on the arm and say something like, "I have confidence in you, I know you can do it", or "Good job, keep up the good work!" Something encouraging. These breakfast meetings left me feeling exhilarated to confused, but for the most part, not down.

    Case, another partner, was the brains of the operation, if there was one. Except he had nothing to with what was going on. He was involved in major meeting with me and Ed once every other month. At one of these meetings, Case got angry at me because the money picture had disintegrated without him finding out about it. He rarely asked for financial information, but he knew about the cash flow problem. I did not feel like I could turn around and blame Ed, so I took it. I was angry at Case for a period after that and it might have affected communication. But, there were no direct lines of communcation between me and Case. So it just became another frustating part of the picture.

    Luther, the only black owner, had even less to do with the whole picture. It was my idea to bring him in to help with a Human Rights case against the company. He proceeded to tear me apart in front of this employee. I was very upset about this because I didn't bring him in to work against me, I brought him in to work with me. I talked to both Ed and Luther about how I felt, that the difference had been aired between me and the employee and there was no need to put me down in the situation in front of the employee. And, if that was necessary, to discuss what would be happening with me beforehand so I wouldn't get so hurt by the situation. The result of my communication is that Ed told Luther that I should run the next meeting instead of Luther.

    I am a very hard boss with myself. I will and can make myself feel very guilty. I guess you would say I am a perfectionist. I will work till the cows come home to get something done, not only so my boss won't criticize me, but so that I can feel "okay" leaving work or about myself.

    In summary on authority, in most cases with bosses, they tell me what to do and I do it well. I feel I am a good communicator. The relationship is usually a good one, unfortunately, in retrospect, not always to my benefit. Criticism I hate, especially when I don't deserve it. Can I ask for help from authority? My last job proved that I can. I kept trying and asking until I got them the help they needed, and then they put Luther in to replace me running the supermarket.

Peers. Since there are only two major jobs where I have had peers, I will discuss them separately. Dakota Packing Company: My peers consisted of my brother-in-law, my father's partner's grandson, the aging bookkeeper and the soon-to-be general manager. The "relatives" all worked together very well. The only competition or talk behind each other's back involved who was getting paid the most The general manager worked well with me when we had to, but we really didn't have a lot to do with each other. He has a vicious temper and I try to steer clear of those type of people unless I have to. Lou, the bookkeeper, and I were in constant competition. We also worked together very well as a team. We had a few angry moments, I think, basically over who was boss. It was the boss's son versus the bookkeeper of twenty years. He was very old fashioned, computer illiterate and not able to move on. Besides, my father did not like him very much. I, on the other hand, wanted to learn, advance and computerize that office. My friend, Jim, and I had been talking about the fact that the person running the office should know how to program the computer for it. That idea paved the way to Lou's retiring and me taking over the office computer system. After nine months at home and part at work, it was finished. I invited Lou out to my house to give him a lesson on the new machine. He decided to retire shortly thereafter. I don't think I maliciously tried to get rid of Lou, but the jury is still out.

Hallmark Pool Corporation: The peers there were salesmen. Working together with them was extremely difficult. They didn't want to listen to a word I said as far as their credit limits or sales. Maybe in a redeeming way, since I left Hallmark, those salesmen took over the company. Last I heard, they went bankrupt. Personally, the salesmen and I got along fine. But, they were sneaky! I tried to compete with them, wage war with them, but unfortunately, the president of the company, at that time, was also a salesman and usually sided with the salesmen.

Subordinates. Yes, I can certainly delegate authority. I believe, though, in treating others as I would like to be treated, I use "please" and "thank-you" as often as possible. I believe in motivating an employee and teaching him or her. Manipulation is a tactic I have used when it was either fire someone or make them want to quit. Unemployment is usually the drawing card here. I thrive, though, on employees learning and taking responsibility. Unfortunately, not all want to do that. I am careful with criticism of employees and I try to tell them in such a way that they understand and are hurt the least. Firing is also something I treat as delicately as possible and is extremely hard for me to do. I know how it feels. But, I will do it.

Am I an analytical person? Yes! I have programmed computers, balanced many general ledgers and besides, I think very logically.

Am I an innovative worker? Yes! At Dakota Packing there was a large accident (workers' compensation) rate of at least four accidents a month. Insurance costs were quite high. I went to work with the help of a couple of insurance companies and fellow workers to develop a working safety program. I thought of the idea of winning a safety game, that would help employees "think safety". A safety manual was written with detail and meaning. Then came the job of selling it. That involved talking in front of fifty employees explaining the program. This happened more than once. Also, because the safety director had to make it work. Well, it worked cutting accidents down to one or two per month and expenses by $60,000 per year. Also, to have an accountant on the job, programming the computer is another example of my innovation.

Are you a creative person? Yes! I have been writing poetry and short stories for years; I hope they get put together in a book someday. I am creative in my work, as I hope you can see.

How I fit on the population curve has been a difficult question to answer. It brings me to a confession I am a manic-depressive. I have been hospitalized three times. Once for severe depression, once for psychotic behavior and the last for manic-depression. I guess I am telling you this because that is a part of what makes me who I am.

Analyzing myself as an introvert or an extrovert is difficult. These are my conclusions. In a social situation I am very much an introvert because of the fact that I find it difficult to be myself when being myself is not socially acceptable. On a one-to-one basis, socially, I can be more extroverted because, I think, I can control the conversation better and I feel more understood. I can also pick who it is I am speaking to. In the workplace, I can be both extroverted and introverted, but I think it is easier for me to joke and be myself at work because, for the most part, people leave their personal lives at home. Besides, being the boss, I can pick and choose what I say or don't say.

November 5, 1991

'TIS THE DAY BEFORE
I BEGIN TO END
A TEST MY LIFE
JUST CAN'T DEPEND.

AHEAD LIES A CHANCE
I'VE BEEN WAITING FOR
TO BE MYSELF
WITH FAMILY & FRIENDS.

AMERICAN BUSINESS TODAY

I need a job to keep me going.
I feel pain most of the time.
Real jobs are impossible to find.
Salesmen as bosses? You're out of your mind!

Unemployment, the fastest growing business,
Not enough to fill the void of employment.
If luck finds me back in the rat race,
I'll need to start looking for a better place.

The economy is supposedly the reason,
There is no chance of finding a job.
Let's look at the way businesses are run,
Too busy worrying about fun in the sun.

Ever been backstabbed while trying to work?
Makes one quite unhappy, enough to quit.
Leaving you looking for a righteous company,
Come on, do you think that could ever be?

Honesty should be such a divine quality.
One should get an award for being that way.
In business you do; they use you and say,
Sucker of the year! Honesty does not pay.

WAITING - 1991

YOU KNOW I HATE TO WAIT,
BUT, IT'S ONLY A DAY NOW.
WAITING MAKES ME FEEL DEPRESSED.
BUT, THERE'S A GOOD CHANCE THIS TIME.
I FEAR I'LL BE REJECTED.
YOU'VE DONE THE BEST YOU CAN.
MAYBE THAT'S NOT GOOD ENOUGH.
THEN, MAYBE IT WASN'T MEANT TO BE.
YOU SEEM TO HAVE ALL THE ANSWERS.
THAT'S BECAUSE I'VE BEEN WATCHING YOU.
ALRIGHT, I FEEL BETTER,
BUT, I STILL HAVE TO WAIT.

THE LEAVES ARE TURNING.
SOON TO BE FALLING.
HOW CAN ONE DECIDE
WHETHER WORK IS CHOSEN BETTER
FROM THE HEART OR FROM THE MIND?
SEEMINGLY, THE ANSWER LIES IN NEED
TO FILL THE TABLES THAT CARE FOR YOUNG.
WHICH KEEP OUR LIVES WHERE THEY BELONG.
BUT, WHAT OF HAPPINESS & FULFILLMENT,
BRINGING MEANING TO OUR LIVES?

I'VE TAKEN THE WRONG PATH
AND DON'T KNOW WHAT IS RIGHT.
THEY SAY, "WHAT DO YOU WANT TO BE?"
LIKE THE ANSWER'S ON THE TIP OF MY TONGUE.
IF I KNEW, THEN THEY COULDN'T BE ASKING,
FOR I WOULD BE THERE; AND THEY WOULD BE HERE.

11/12/91 - MANSFIELD, NEW JERSEY

"WHY? WHY DID YOU DO IT? I CAN'T BELIEVE YOU DID THAT!"

"I DIDN'T MEAN TO DO IT. I WAS ONLY TRYING TO HELP."

THE WORDS AND THOUGHTS OF A PARENT AND CHILD WHEN THINGS JUST AREN'T WORKING OUT. I'VE BEEN ON BOTH SIDES OF THIS ISSUE. HERE ARE TWO POEMS WRITTEN WITH THE FEELINGS I HAVE FELT AND BECAME HELPLESS TO DO ANYTHING ABOUT.

THE CHILD
MOMMY AND DADDY ARE MY IDOLS.
I LOVE THEM SO MUCH.
I WANT TO BE WITH THEM;
EVERYDAY AND IN EVERYWAY.

I KEEP WAITING FOR MY FATHER,
TO COME HOME FROM WORK.
HE SPENDS TIME WITH ME,
WHILE HE WATCHES SPORTS ON T.V.

I LIE ON ONE COUCH, IN OUR FAMILY ROOM,
AND HE ON THE OTHER IN THE VERY SAME ROOM,
READING HIS NEWSPAPER; WHICH ACTED AS A FENCE.
DISTURBING HIM, I FEAR, MAKES VERY LITTLE SENSE.

I just had a job where, at times,
I was happier while I was unemployed.
You see, control is such a major issue,
Despite success, they fire and won't miss you.

I sure would like to trust a boss.
You can't, of course, it's not a choice.
Whatever happened to people working as one,
That's the only way that things get done.

FEBRUARY 1992

BEING OVERPROTECTED AND IGNORED,
CAN KILL YOU.
BUT, THERE IS NO SENTENCE
FOR THIS HEINOUS CRIME.
NO BLAME FOR DAMAGE DONE,
ONLY GUILT.

10/31/93

They say you can do it.
But, I can't, I hurt too bad.
You've only got three days to go.
I don't want to study anymore.
You want your C.P.A., don't you?
Yes but this is too much to take.
Push yourself, it will be worth it.
It's not that I don't want to,
I just don't feel like it.
Then stop, give it up, quit.
Don't be so hard on me.
I want to feel good when this over.
Just give it your best shot,
And all anyone can say. is you did the best you could.
That's bullshit because we both know,
That succeeding is what I'm in this for.
Not the effort or the pain.
I'm trying, but don't expect glee from me!

6/12/94

When the words and the actions
Don't go together,
What kind of message are we sending?
If we believe any part,
We will see what we want,
While the truth be not known by any.

6/27/94

Friendship is the give and take of love without the need for a committment.

July 17, 1994

07:37 AM

Why do I need the warmth of a woman?
Why do I need her when I am alone?
When she's not there, I'm not here.
When I'm not here, I get lost.

I naturally depend on one for all,
But, I've learned that friends can make me strong.
Her love is so much a part of me.
When she's away, it's hard to be free.

Her life's not mine right now.
I don't know if it will ever be.
Do I believe her words of love?
Is it enough to know how much we care?

We seem to hold on to ups and downs,
Happiness is such a foreign word.
Together, we can be free,
Alone, it's just you and me.

8:27 A.M.

8:37 A.M.

Waiting is not my favorite thing,
In fact, I really hate it.
My life's too short this time,
To wait for what I need.

8:44 A.M.

She says I'm a role model.
I say she's a role model.
What a joke we make.
It takes the cake.

The answer is to wait,
And never be late,
Because I don't have any dates,
And I lost my two mates.

It's eight thirty seven,
I'll stay up till eleven.
If I can make it that far,
I'll be shooting par.

Maybe it's just fate,
That I need to wait.
So for G-d's sake,
Go jump in a lake.

I don't play games.

7/24/94-9:08 P.M.

Why can't we see what will be,
I need to feel the future.
To know what my outcome must be,
Would lighten my load, for sure.

Roses are red,
Violets are green.
If Tammy doesn't marry me,
I know I will scream.

Arthur Andersen LLP
33 West Monroe Street
Chicago, IL 6063

October 10, 1994

Dear David:

Congratulations on passing the CPA exam! This is a significant accomplishment and something that you should be proud of. The outside world values this designation, and it's something that you will carry with you always.

Congratulations again.

Dean

Mr. David Samuelson
Arthur Andersen LLP
33 West Monroe Street
Chicago, Illinois 60603

10/22/94

I never wanted to hurt you, Tammy.
There was just too much pain choosing between.
Why couldn't we have been well and single,
Or the loss of our friendship been foreseen.

Lettice & Lovage—11/94

They say kids always want to play,
Playing again was this kid's dream.

First Change

1. Hat off
2. Pipe out of coat pocket
3. Coat off
4. Ring off

Second Change

1. Turtleneck off (untuck first)
2. Tuck in tee shirt
3. Glasses out of case and on
4. Pipe into case in back pocket
5. Hand thru hair
6. Close Door

1/15/95-2:00 A.M.

Being down is shading my life,
Can anything help to ease my strife?
I work hard to keep myself up.
Others take strength to fill their cup.
Why not me?

3/16/95

I can't believe it. After all this time, I am finally free. From what you ask? Well it may not seem like much to you, but, I don't know how to explain it. Okay, let me try.

I am forty years young. I am also a manic-depressive. I believe I have had this ailment for just about every one of those years. I wrote my first poem about depression when I was just twelve years old. Do you see how hard this is to explain? How can I tell you what it's been like for me? Better yet, how can I help you to understand what it's like now to suddenly lose all the remaining symptoms of my illness?

March 21, 1995

2:30 AM

And then it all changed. I don't understand it, but everything is different. I can think. I can see. I can hear. I can love.

What happens now? I'm finally walking man's road. Which way do I go? I'm scared.

So, I write; something I've done many nights before. It seems the same to me, like it always has. But, maybe it's not. Perhaps my words make more sense now.

I haven't written very many words tonight. It's not been my way for a long time. I guess I've written in dribs and drabs, in spurts.

I need to be constant. I need to keep my base. I need to move forward, but oh how that tears at my heart. I've lived in such fear of life, of people, of myself.

I have waited for this day. I have prayed for this day. Now that it's here, I don't know what to do.

I can't sleep but I need to sleep. Tomorrow is coming. I have to relax, forget all this. Can I do that? Who's stopping me? I am. I have been my own worst enemy all along and it seems like that hasn't changed. I guess I'll just lay down and think of fairy tales, like I always have. I'll drink some *hot chocolate,* too. I've been listening to soothing music, after all.

This could really work. Just me, myself, and I as a team. I'm alive!

March 31, 1995

3:00 A.M.

> Popularity breeds contempt.
> Do you really want to hurt me?
> How can anybody be so cruel?
> Boy George

You are mentally ill, that is why you are doing this. You lose jobs in the fall and this happened last year same time. It's all cyclical. Yon really need to think about this. I'm just trying to be your friend. Nobody knows you better than I do.

Then I defend myself.

If that's true what do you want with a mentally ill person? If you do, you need to get your head examined. You're not my friend. You knew me then, you don't know me now. If you were my friend and really knew me, you wouldn't try to hurt me in this way. You were born with no empathy at all. You hit someone and expect them to thank you for caring. I also pointed out job inaccuracies. Cyclical in that you called me mentally ill last year too!

I refuse to be treated like this anymore.

Our world needs to knock on wood,
While treating life just as we should.
Dying and living,
Lying and forgiving,
Are guided by faith,
In what G-d sayeth.

Chapter 7

5/3/95 - Tammy's words on the answering machine

Thank you for embracing the love that I give to you. It brings me much joy and fulfillment. I feel that our relationship has opened up like a stream that has been freed up after very long restrictions. Now love, truth and hope flow freely and infinitely with a peacefulness beyond explanation. Your love has put the life back into my soul. Thank you and I love you!

Some inspirational things that might help! Stuart Smalley: Fear is a darkroom where negatives get developed. From a book: Hope is the lantern of the soul. Nothing can defeat you unless you surrender. Visualize the good, believe the good, accept the good. Hope is a sweet expectation that never sleeps. Fear is only the absense of belief. You cannot know your strength until you test it. The love we give to others returns to bring us joy.

May 7, 1995

08:51 AM

The challenges life presents me,
Are mind boggling right now.
A divorce, possible lack of job,
A suicidal girlfriend,
Living in the same house as my soon to be ex-wife.
Is there anything else that could happen to make it worse?
Oh yes, the dream I had today,
About my wife telling me off for divorcing her,
And me actually believing that she might be right.
Do I stay here?
I can't leave my girlfriend now!
Where do I pursue a job?
Can I make it?
Thank God I see Fred tomorrow,
Because I need a shot in the arm.
Dear Diary, I love Tammy!

Tammy
5/27/95 11:00 P.M.

If I can't speak,
I have to write.
My thoughts center in one place.
All around the features of a face.
The love of my life.
I'd give my left nut to be with you now.
Then when you were in Omni,
You could see it next to the rest of the nuts.
Without you, I'm alone.
Your memory keeps me whole,
Even if I only have one nut.
Did I tell you I'm nuts about you?
So I'm a dirt bag and a weirdo, huh?
I'm sure glad you got you're 80 cents worth.
Well, this weird dirt bag is madly in love with you.
You can call me anything you want.
But, I would never sink so low to call you names, you douche bag.
I feel so good loving you.
I don't deserve someone as good as you.
I'm the luckiest guy in the world,
And I can't forget that.
I want you more than anything in this whole world.
I love you so much.
You're the best there is.

6/17/95

Pain is not something to be measured.
Pain is something to be cared for.

9/95

What do I do?
My options are few.
I've made my bed,
Now I wish I was dead.

It's an upward climb,
But I don't have time.
I need to find,
What I left behind.

I can pretend I'm someone I'm not,
It helps a little, but not a lot.
Please stop hurting me,
But why just let me be.

I want to see Bread,
With the person that I wed.
I'm enjoying the pain,
I guess I can't complain.

March 31, 1996

02:00 - 3:00 AM

And now I'm alone.
No one to care for,
Except myself and the phone.
Can't you see that I need more?

Where to turn, how to find,
The answer that's not inside.
How did I get in to this bind?
Will I ever stem the tide?

Wait they say; there's pain I say.
I've been alone for far too long.
How much do I have to pay,
To save my life from all that's wrong?

The time will come.
I feel it near.
I must be numb.
This is my year.

June 16, 1996

11:30 PM

A hurt can twist so deep,
That words won't make it sleep.
You live each day in pain.
It makes you feel insane.

What manner of peace is there,
When love is all but rare?
The hurt whirls round the lack of this,
And something as simple as a kiss.

I need this love I've never had,
To make me whole and oh so glad.
Will it come sometime this life?
Don't worry, I won't end it with a knife.

June 17, 1996

03:15 AM

It won't go away.
No matter how hard I try,
I can't forget that time,
When life could make me cry.

Now the tears don't come.
I guess I'm just numb.
I'm tired of that hurtful life,
So filled with heartache and strife.

Please, let me leave it behind.
I need to be with my kind.
I can't afford to be blind.
I've made up my mind.

June 19, 1996

07:45 PM

Pain, pain, go away,
Come again some other day.

Waiting for the phone to ring,
Is really not my kind of thing.
Where have all the people gone?
I scared them away.

My stomach says I have to eat.
I can't, you see, I'm in retreat.

You see, I'm lost,
Forget the cost.
Who am I?
I need to cry.

Someone find me sitting here,
And squeeze away this awful fear.

Why do I pick my eyebrows?

July 25, 1996

10:57 AM

Another friend is moving away,
And though I'd rather that you stay,
Finally here's your chance to be free,
And become what you really want to be.

I will miss the perfect timing,
While the laughter keeps on climbing.
You will bless others with your gift,
While memories will give me a lift.

We seem to understand each other,
And I know we will find another,
To be our friend through thick and thin,
Very much like you've always been.

You believed in me,
And helped me to be,
More than I ever knew,
I could be without you.

Please don't lose touch with me.
We can both be free.
We can continue to grow while apart,
While your still in my heart.

Happy Birthday, Mom!
Hope sixty is happy!

If flies could speak
what would they say,
To those of us who dash and seek
For weapons; then kill them everyday.

May 11, 1997

12:30 AM

Can't see; don't even want to.
Fear has gripped me through and through,
With nothing to hold onto except me,
And I thought I needed to break free.

Friends have come like before,
Always leaving me with no score.
My strength is dependent on,
What I thought I had; now gone.

Respect others and they will respect you,
Doesn't work in this animal zoo.
Survival of the fittest rings true.
Honesty and sensitivity certainly won't do.

7/2/97 5:00 P.M. (on the train)

I'm almost there.
Boy I'm scared.
I feel it near,
Filled with fear.
Can't turn back.
What do I lack?
So close now.
Don't know how.
Have no choice.
I hear a voice.

August 10, 1997

05:20 AM

Life is upon me,
And it's almost too much.
But now I can see.
If only I could touch.

It's hard to sleep.
My thoughts run deep.
I seem so close.
I don't need another dose.

I've been this close before,
But never through that door.
Somehow I must go on.
I need love to keep me strong.

Loneliness is hard for me.
Somehow there lies the key,
To unlock the fears inside.
There's no place left to hide.

August 13, 1997

10:15 PM

Dear Anna,

As usual, I can't get the thought of you out of my mind. So, I thought I would write you and send you some positive energy. If you were here I would probably be talking with you right now. But don't feel bad. I am happy that you can spend some time in Poland.

I got the Emerson, Lake and Palmer tickets today. We won't be able to see very well, but it will sound great!

Have I told you lately how beautiful you are? Well, you are! And don't you forget it. The thoughts of you brighten my life. You put a smile on my face throughout the day.

I hope you are having a good time. I hope your flight was a good one. I hope that everybody is doing fine.

I went for a walk with Donna, my next door neighbor. It was good to get some exercise and also to have someone to talk to. She's really a fine person. You'll have to meet her someday.

So, you want poetry, huh? Well this will have to be right off the top of my head.

> I feel a change coming on,
> And it's not because you're gone.
> It's because you are in my heart.
> Could this be just the start?

It's time for me to get ready to try to sleep tonight. I will write you again soon.

Love, David

8/15/97 10:15 P.M.
8/16/97 12:15 A.M.

I'm afraid of getting hurt.
If shunned, I'll feel like dirt.
I love someone I don't know.
She's inside me wherever I go.

My sensitivity scares my past.
I feel fear; the die is cast.
Even if you're not the last.
Anna, my dear, my love came fast.

I need to know more about you.
Our talks are short; our meetings few.
My wish is to fulfill our dreams.
That's always harder than it seems.

August 17, 1997

04:30 AM

"Why? Why? Why can't I be like everyone else?" he whispered softly aloud. Abe didn't know. But, that's what he wanted more than anything else in this world.

It was a beautiful day. The sun was shining and the birds were chirping. He could hear the muted voices of children playing. The date was Friday, June 13, 1997. Abe had pulled all the shades closed in the house. He did not want to see the day, nor the day to see him.

His easy chair was at an angle facing the stereo. That's funny, he thought, I'm facing the music. He chuckled quietly at his own joke. He was alone. He lived by himself in a condominium on the first floor. He had called in sick to work that day. He didn't like this day.

Abe got up out of his easy chair and walked slowly into the kitchen. He opened the refrigerator and took out a bottle of apple juice. Unscrewing the top, he put the liquid to his mouth and drank at least three gulps. He put the bottle back and returned to his comfort zone.

The music kept on changing tempo. That was his choice; he had on a variety of CD's. He loved his music. It could make him forget, at times, his unhappiness and his loneliness.

The telephone rudely arrested his thoughts. Abe jumped up to check his "Caller I.D.". "Unknown" was what he saw. That usually meant that someone wanted to sell him something. But, he knew he had to pick up the phone, since work was also "Unknown". He let the phone ring one more time, then slowly picked up the telephone.

August 21, 1997

07:55 AM

"Hello", he said in a sickly voice.

"Hello", replied a familiar voice. Abe couldn't quite place the voice, but he knew it.

"How are you?" asked Abe.

"The same", answered the voice.

Who was this? It was killing him because the person sounded so familiar. It almost sounded like his father, but his father was dead. What should he do?

"How are you?" questioned the presence on the other end of the phone.

"I'm sick today", said Abe, unsure of himself, but knowing exactly how he was feeling.

Suddenly Abe heard a click in the telephone attached to his hand and then a quick dial tone.

August 24, 1997

11:17 PM

Dear Anna,

You're still on my mind constantly. I so look forward to you coming home. I hope you feel that I am someone to come home to.

Words cannot describe how beautiful and special you are to me. I love talking with you. You are so smart.

I hope I receive a letter from you before you get back. Everyday's high point for me is the possibility that a letter from you might be in my mailbox.

I could tell you about the business, but I'll tell you all about it when you get back. A week from today, I will hopefully have talked to you. I hope you are having a good time and that you can come back rested and refreshed.

I miss you and I want you back sooner then you are actually arriving. But, I am doing well. It's still hard to sleep sometimes. Between the business and you, I've got a lot on my mind. I hope somehow you can receive this message telepathically, because I'm not going to mail it. But you will see (hear) it when you get back.

I think about your son, also. He seems like such a good kid and I look forward to getting to know him better. I told my son about Great America today. We spent the day together. He's excited about it.

Enjoy your last week in Poland. I will talk to you soon.

Love,
Dave

August 26, 1997

10:20 PM

Dear Anna,

I'm almost as far as I can go with my business preparations. I'm negotiating the franchise agreement. I've found a location and I will finish my business plan tonight and tomorrow.

I miss you. I miss your kind words and your beautiful face. I feel very comfortable around you. You're coming home in five days. I hope we care about each other. I hope we want to talk to each other. But, all I can do is hope.

I think it was love at first sight. I didn't believe in that until I saw you. Enjoy your remaining time in Poland. Talk to you soon.

Love,
Dave

P.S. Did you write me?

August 28, 1997

11:30 PM

Dear Anna,

I can't sleep thinking about you. I'm so happy that you are coming home. I got your postcard yesterday and it filled me with joy. Thank you.

I finished my business plan yesterday. I also found a location and am negotiating my franchise agreement. You were very important in all this happening. With you behind me, I can do anything.

Have I mentioned how beautiful you are? Don't get tired of it, because I can't help but speak the truth. I am counting the days till I will hear from you. I hope I'm not overdoing it. I feel the way I feel. And if I get hurt because of this, it certainly will not be the first time. And it will not be the last. I think I am in love with you. Can you believe that? It's hard for me, but I know the feeling. I want to hug you and kiss you. Enough! Until I speak with you on Sunday.

Love,
David

August 29, 1997

10:45 PM

My sweet Anna,
I'd like to peel you like a banana.

October 26, 1997

01:45 AM

Where I am, What I've done,
And even the lack of fun.
I have my friends to thank,
For helping me succeed at the bank.

But that's only a minor point.
It's been like having an extra joint,
To pull me through the tough times,
When, at times, nothing seemed to rhyme.

There's Anna, my brave psychologist,
Who gave me strength to make a fist.
Kathy, my rigid backbone,
Who believed in me while on the phone.

Larry, whose faithfulness helped me,
To be what I knew I could be.
Judy, who told me what I needed to hear,
In order for me to see my fear.

Tammy, my loyal friend,
I know we will be together till the end.
There is more than that, I know.
To you my gratitude for helping me grow.

To my mother, I feel sorry for her.
She felt the need to try to deter.
She needs to grow up along with me.
Only then will she ever have a chance to see.

Now I'm scared to sign the lease.
I hope my best will bring me peace.
My hat is off to those who believe in me,
Without you I could never feel free.

November 28, 1997

04:42 AM

I don't have a family.
They all just flee,
Or push me away,
And that's where they'll stay.

I have my work cut out for me,
To build my life so I can be,
Fulfilled, respected and important.
Something I've only experienced as an infant.

I'm on the right path.
I don't need any fancy math.
I just need love in my life.
I promise I won't destroy my next wife.

January 18, 1998

11:03 PM

The tide flows in.
It also flows out.
Life continues within,
As it continues without.

The passage of time has changed things.
I no longer wear wedding rings.
I stand alone stronger then ever,
Looking for someone to make me feel better.

Patience is still the key,
That separates me from what I could be.
Maybe someday I will see,
How to wait, thus pay the fee.

I don't need to be disappointed again,
Nor feel more pain entering in.
I want to trust and I must,
But somehow I still can't get through the crust.

So I sit on my couch wondering,
What will come next; excitement or fear.
As always, something neither black or white.
I need someone to help me fight.

The tide flows in.
It also flows out.
Life continues within,
As it continues without.

March 30, 1998

12:30 AM

If you do something wrong,
You can see it on their face.
Why do you keep looking at me?
There could never be enough space.

I can't see this year,
And maybe not the next.
I'm afraid of you; you see.
Please, stay in your place.

September 7, 1998

01:30 AM

This time is strange.
I know it not.
My health is here.
My friends are not.

David - I am very, very, very, very depressed. I can not change the past. I have destroyed the rest of my life, why not this too. I am a loser. Go somewhere where you can be unconditionally taken care of, because I fucked up!

Paula - You said that I did not have a life, but that you had CD Warehouse. You said you made a mistake in all our dreams and you said you did not know if we could have a relationship at all. You said it so final. Of course, you were at work which makes it hard, but you really acted like you were through with me last weekend. What would anyone else think? I was devastated by your firmness and you never called again. I even said I loved you but you said nothing at all.

David - You have to choose what to believe.

Paula - Dave, if you were afraid once, you could be afraid again. I'm so lost in this I can't even trust myself anymore. Four days of emptiness was almost too much to take. I'm confused as to what to do! I'm so hurt and messed up. It's going to take forever to fix my life. Lost in lost world.

David - If this relationship is going to work, I have to understand anxiety. I don't right now and that is why I was confused and I ran for my life. I want to accept and understand you, but you have to give me a chance.

Paula - We should all go on "The Jerry Springer Show"!

Dear David,

    This is for you. Have a great day!

    Play the side ready to play—there's a short delay between the 2 songs.

Love,
Paula

February 10, 1999

02:15 AM

Your pain is my pain.
My pain is your pain.
I've never met a woman,
Who completes me like you do.

I fear you will leave me,
Like the others in my life.
You are afraid I will flee.
I love you so much, can't you see?

Our lives are full of strife.
When you someday become my wife.
Your inner beauty will shine for me,
And I will finally be able to see.

We both have shed tears,
Throughout our many years.
Faintly I hear the cheers,
While we wrestle with our fears.

You are more important to me,
Then anything else could be.
My fears speak out so loudly,
That my love appears cloudy.

So, how do we cope,
With our many fears?
Love is the answer,
And all I ever want is you.

2/10/99 9:20 A.M.

Hurting you is like hurting myself.
My life is connected to yours.

Chapter 8

Rockford - Hospital Stay - 1999

March 26—4:15 Checked In CDH
March 26—7:38 Checked in Rockford
March 27—Today
March 28—Tomorrow
March 29—The Day After That
March 30—2 mo. until Jesse's B'day
March 31—Donna & Mike's Anniversary
April 1—April Fool's Day
April 2—Day after April Fool's Day
April 3—Some people still thinking it's April Fool's Day

Secrets to Happiness

Here are a list of secrets to happiness from a recent Quaker newsletter:

- *Live beneath your means.*
- *Return everything you borrow.*
- *Stop blaming other people.*
- *Admit it when you make a mistake.*
- *Give clothes not worn in 3 years to charity.*
- *Do something nice and try not to get caught.*
- *Listen more; talk less.*
- *Every day take a 30-minute walk.*
- *Strive for excellence, not perfection.*
- *Be on time.*
- *Don't make excuses.*
- *Don't argue.*
- *Get organized.*
- *Be kind to kind people.*
- *Be even kinder to unkind people.*
- *Let someone cut ahead of you in line.*
- *Take time to be alone.*
- *Reread a favorite book.*
- *Cultivate good manners.*
- *Be humble.*
- *Realize and accept that life isn't always fair.*
- *Know when to say something.*
- *Know when to keep your mouth shut.*
- *Go an entire day without criticizing anyone.*
- *Learn from the past.*
- *Plan for the future.*
- *Live in the present.*
- *Don't sweat the small stuff.*
- *It's all small stuff.*

March 26, 1999

11:21 PM

I'm in Rockford, what a treat.
If only I could meet on the street.
Kindly pass by someone without hurting intent,
Unfortunately makes for a situation.

I'm in Rockford, what a treat,
If only I could meet on the street.
The Session has started.
All the people and children.

March 30, 1999

05:54 PM

When it seems like the whole world is against you,
And there's no one to turn to who knows you better than you.
What do you do?
What do you say?
How can you exist?
I know how.
Grin and bear it.
Things always get worse before they get better.
Hold out.
Stand fast.
Things will work out in the end.
The question is,
Why not now?

List everything you worry about—big things, little things, anything that causes you concern or makes you uneasy.

1. Personal Health
2. Being Comfortable
3. Keeping my Job
4. Where do I go after I die
5. Equal Rights between Men and Women

In different relationships we decide the balance between "public" and "private" self quite differently. No one should share themselves equally with everyone. But if you share yourself with no one, your overall health is likely to suffer.

What are you willing to share (public self) with your . . .	What are you not willing to share (private self)?
1. Spouse – Everything	Nothing
2. Children – Almost Everything	Sex
3. Parents—Almost Nothing	Everything
4. Best Friend – Everything	Nothing
5. Work Associates – Superficial	Personal Beliefs

To what degree is your "public self" different from your "private self"? I'd like them to be the same, but intelligence stops me.

What kinds of things have you never shared with anyone? The truth about my parents.

How does your self-disclosure differ with men and with women? Why? More disclosure to women. Women are easier to get to know and trust.

Lina

I had an Oma Lina once.
She was kind and sweet and Henry's mother.
The biggest problem with Oma Lina,
Was the fact that she was so short,
And very very wrinkled.
My Lina is a thing of beauty.
Honest, straightforward, gorgeous, and petite.
The question is, how do I tell her,
The way I feel about her.
My Lina . . .

April 5, 1999

TWENTY THINGS I LOVE TO DO
1. Act
2. Be with children
3. Run
4. Play Games
5. Drive
6. Listen to Music
7. Ride a Train
8. Ride a Plane
9. Take Vacations
10. Make Love
11. Fall in Love with the Right Person
12. Get Help for my Mental Illness
13. Look at Women
14. Shop for Music
15. Shop for Autographs
16. Public Speak
17. Talk to People
18. Fix Things Around the House
19. Clean the House
20. Not Talk to my Mother

After you have completed the section above, ask yourself what you have learned.

1. I learned that everything requires planning.
2. I learned I like to do more things with someone else.
3. I learned I like to do least things alone.

Nontraditional leisure activities often are non-structured.

1. Jigsaw Puzzles
2. Getting an "A" on an exam I didn't study for.

What do you find yourself doing when you are bored?
1. Watch T.V.
2. Read

What emotions do you feel when you are bored?
1. Lonely
2. Sad
3. Detached

What seems to help you get out of feeling bored?
1. People

Boredom comes from: Being Alone

Values are the roots of the leisure decisions we make. What is a value?
1. Something worth a lot to us.

What is a natural high?
1. Rocky Mountain High, Colorado

Write a list of your personal natural highs.
1. Listening to "America"
2. Listening to "Argent"
3. Listening to "The Beatles"
4. Listening to "Russ Ballard"
5. Listening to "The Zombies"
6. Listening to "Colin Blunstone"
7. Making Love
8. Playing with the Kids
9. Going to Football Games
10. Going to Basketball Games

The one thing that I learned most about myself and my leisure lifestyle through this program is: All Work and no Play makes David a Dull Boy. Additional Comments about this program: Thank-you!

Bi - Pola*roïd*

They were first cousins, but they loved.
They were innocent yet they sinned.
Their male offspring suffered greatly with an illness.
Now all that's left of that illness is me and my son.
What can we become?
We will become the best that we can be.
Computers for my son.
Who knows what's for me.
Time will tell the truth.
Mood swings may come and go,
But the person inside remains the same,
But we have to convince people we are tame!

The End

The hospital is beautiful.
Not to say the other wasn't.
But, the compassion and understanding,
Displayed by these brave people,
Put them in a true place of honor.
And Don't You Forget it!
I love anyone who respects, cares, & understands me.
I love my cousins.
I love my aunt & uncles.
I love you Dad!
I especially love Kyle.
I love you Larry.
I love you Gail.
I love you Terrie!
I love you Jessica!
I love you Sue!
I love you Tammy!
I love my kids.
I love my mother.
I love my sister's family.
I love you Judy.
That's—That's—That's all Folks!

THE END

April 10, 1999

05:35 PM

The Beginning of the End of this Book.

March 4, 2000

She moves like a dream,
You wish she'd wear ice cream,
Although it's cold, you know.
She was there, bearing gifts.
And coy, yes, very coy.
Stop kidding yourself.
I love you, so there; okay?
Where have you gone, who knows?

March 4, 2000

'Tis really a bore,
But, what do I care.
I hear the music from far.
He's coming in, do I give a damn?!

March 5, 2000

02:00 AM

Could this all be true?
My music has caught on with a few.
And I feel more open to life.
What I need today is a wife.
Where does one look for this,
Or something as allusive as a kiss.
I'll wait for the right lady.
Pleasure for me would be having a baby,
To care for through thick and thin.
I'll always wonder, where has she been?

April 29, 2000

10:15 PM

Time keeps passing by,
While life stays the same.
I'm not afraid of change,
It's just, how do I get there?

I know. I can do it now.
Patience has been my friend,
I've needed it to mend,
Fractures; this can't be my last bow.

Now I write to heal,
My next rollercoaster ride.
I'm still screaming from the last.
I've got to be smart, unlike the past.

And again I'm alone,
But not depressed; always thinking.
I'm so smart, I know that,
It scares people, but not me.

April 30, 2000

08:25 PM

I've just been out with my maker.
It was fun, challenging and breath taking.
When we said goodbye, I said I love you.
She said me too.
I'd have to be to put up with you,
All these years.

May 10, 2000

06:35 PM

I feel so shy and timid, because you know,
I'll only get hurt again.
Why should I even pretend.
That she's the one for me.

May 13, 2000

04:00 PM

He sits alone in his living room hide away, listening to music from the soundtrack to his favorite movie. Alone. No not alone. His cat, Lady, is sitting cleaning herself, but still watching him, he knows.

He begins to think about the recent past that has again put him in his place. He's trying. It's just that it's not his time yet. He knows that, but lingers through some sad feelings.

On Thursday, he locked his keys in the car with the motor running. After physical therapy, still in his sweat suit, he went to the supermarket. Having no pockets, he was very conscious of carrying his checkbook in his hand. By the time he got to the checkout stand, a crushing thought blew him away.

June 10, 2000

09:34 PM

What will I do with the rest of my life? Once a loser, always a loser. Right? I'm listening to "Philadelpia Freedom". It's inspired by Billie Jean King. I feel hopeless. No one will ever care for me again or even about me. Writing is painful. I think too much; see too little in the future.

June 11, 2000

09:50 PM

I'm like an open sore.
I need some luck right now,
Or I'll be on the floor.
Keep going and close my mouth,
Is my only avenue,
Since I can't handle people.
No matter what they say or do,
It's like a knife in my ego.
I'll try to keep it together,
Until this "Twilight Zone" ends.

June 12, 2000

10:53 PM

I can't find the words.

June 23, 2000`

10:35 PM

Realization has made things clear.
Can I withstand the feeling of fear?
Is this a breakthrough or not?
All I know, this is all I've got.

June 25, 2000

06:50 PM

I'm left alone.
Try the phone.
Watch a "Twilight Zone".
Give the guy a bone.
Oh for a sigh or moan.
This is the life I own.
Feeling better with an ice cream cone?
No, I need a new brain sewn.

June 26, 2000

11:05 PM

I gave away a friend.
Respect was more important.
Logic, not feelings, he could not bend.
Emotion he could taste.

June 30, 2000

I got fired from my job.
Believe me, I will not sob.
They hired me for one thing,
And paid me to do another.
I can do better!

July 14, 2000

Life is temporary, so they say.
As is my work, I'm afraid to say.
It is not so bad, I have to pay.
Sitting around breaks my back any day.

July 23, 2000

3:00 P.M.

(Song)

Please forgive me for being who I am.
An honest guy trying life as a man.
Dealing with highs and lows amidst stigma.
But, don't be afraid, there are ways to learn.
Still I love her and I always will.
You've got to accept the bad with the good.
You are beautiful, meaning well to all.
I'm not yours because of this damn illness.
I will keep on changing throughout my life.
Most of it being good, with a fringe of bad.
My tender heart longing for a true love.
Still I love you and I always will.
You've got to take the bad with the good.
Please forgive me for being who I am,
An honest guy trying life as a man,
So don't be afraid, there are ways to learn.
I love you and I always will.
You've got to take the bad with the good.
My sense of humor brings smiles all around,
Except when depression blinds any laugh.
I think I'm the great communicator.
Sometimes meaningful talk cannot be found.
Still I love her and I always will.
You've got to accept the bad with the good.
She is beautiful, meaning well to all.
I can't be yours due to this damn illnes.
I will keep changing throughout my life,
My tender heart longing for a true Iove.
Still I love her, and I always will.
You've got to accept the bad with the good.

Middle Eight

I still dream of a cure,
Where we are all equal.
Where relatives like us,
And friends don't run away.

August 16, 2000

10:20 PM

Where is it going?
When will it end?
Can I keep going?
Will I defend?
I need so much.
Where do I get it?
I feel so alone.
I need validation!

September 23, 2000

Why are things always the loneliest on Saturday night? I've tried writing this on numerous occasions. It never stuck. So, I will try it again. This time I'll start in the middle. I think that things were as bad then as they are now. What a revelation. Things always go up and down, back and forth; never in and out.

I just rang the phone. Of course, no one's home. It's Saturday night. If I could only write this, my life would have some meaning. Wish me luck. God knows I need it.

September 25, 2000

09:53 PM

I knew I should have written rather than give the stop light to a short story. I started watching a movie, called "Leaving Las Vegas". I fell asleep on it for at least the fourth time. Well, I didn't make it this time either. I fell asleep. Sometimes when I take a nap, I wake up feeling very depressed and paranoid. It almost feels like a very bad hangover. Recovering from these naps is very painful and usually takes between fifteen minutes to an hour. This one was a doozy. I decided to put the movie back on so I could finally see the end. That was a mistake. That movie should never be seen by someone dealing with a depressive illness. I was not helped in the least by watching it. Finally, an hour later, I went to the DMDA (Depressive Manic-Depressive Association) meeting. Still down. Being a manic-depressive (bipolar) is certainly a pain in the ass.

Same Night 10:40 P.M.

All of a sudden, I feel a hypomanic rush to my forehead. Mental illness is a friend to no one. What will I do about it? Whatever, I need to get some sleep. Don't worry, I'll be alright.

Continues (Same Night)

You have no idea how sad I am right now. My life is empty again. Wait . . . let me talk about starting in the middle instead.

I first talked to Terrie around August of 1978. Our conversations were funny and pleasant. Before I would call her, I would always smoke pot. Pot was my way of dealing with loneliness.

I just took a short walk outside. The air is nice. My next door neighbor has her kitchen light on. I've thought of calling her, but I decided not to. Nobody wants to be depressed.

I've switched pens twice since I started writing this. This pen feels comfortable. The color fits my mood (blue). Let's begin. After I was relatively high, I would call. her. It did not take her very long before she poured herself a glass of wine. She normally had two glasses before our conversations were over.

Music. To warm my heart. To undepress my soul. Who better to do that than the Brian Wilson. The beautiful harmonies. Some needed solace.

October 20, 2000

12:00 AM

Before my second marriage, two major idols in my life were Harry Chapin and John Lennon. My ex-wife is a little under eight years older than me. Both of my idols had wives, at that time, that were eight years older than their mates.

The fact that these relationships worked helped convince me that marrying someone as old as Terrie would be a wise thing to do. Not only wise, but a convincing decision making reason.

Unfortunately, after I was married at the end of 1979, both John and Harry were both dead by the Summer of 1981.

October 21, 2000

02:20 PM

Again the depression has lifted.
For how long, G-d only knows.
I hope these poems and stories,
Help you to understand my world.
To boldly go where no man has gone before.
That's the signpost up ahead.
Next stop, the "Twilight Zone".
I feel so much better,
Both physically and mentally.
This will have to be my happy ending.
Life is long, please live it with me.

March 31, 2001. 12:00 A.M.
Frustration

The need for completion,
But not even close.
I have to do it.
You're nothing but dirt.
How do I break the trend?
I want to succeed so badly.
Keep on going; you're only chance.
No promise, you see, please watch.

February 13, 2005 (To my mother)

Whether you want to remember or not,
Today is your seventy-fourth birthday.
Which reminds me, lately I haven't seen you a lot.
And I miss that in a very big way.
So I'd like to see you at least once a month,
For a movie, family get together or such.
And maybe you'll let me pay for the first,
And even a little each month,
You see, I love you and I have lost time with you.
I need to touch.

Chapter 9

The Present

Part 1

I opened my presents with the feeling of conquering the world. I knew what I was going to get, because my wishes to Santa, for 100 years, have been explicit. And besides that, my parents have a lot of money.

The first present was shaped like a triangle with very sharp points and edges. I tore the paper off as fast as I could. Mom and Dad were standing right behind me. Mom had this shit eattin' grin on her face while Dad looked on thinking about the lay he might get tonight if he played his cards right. Finally, the paper was off the present. Lights flashed and bells rang and I knew it was time to go on to my next present. This one was on the inside of a very small box with a pretty blue ribbon on the top. Dad couldn't wait any longer. He grabbed the present for my mother and gave it to her. She opened it with great fervor. It was a necklace with a gold chain and a diamond swinging in the middle about the size of a tennis ball. That was some kiss Mom gave Dad. And now it was Dad who had on that crazy grin.

While all this was going on, my second present was becoming my prey. It was a blow-up bicycle; you know, the kind you blow on one of the pedals and it becomes a big old hairy bike. That's really a nice present, huh? But, I still hadn't gotten what I wanted yet. I wanted one of those gadgets Jimmy Zale plays with all of the time. You have to see it to believe it. You push a button and it gives you all the answers to your homework problems. The blue button is the neatest of them all. I opened my third present and when I saw it, I got that goofy smile on my face.

Just then, the doorbell rang. My Mom and Dad went to answer the door. It was my Uncle Sam and my Aunt Annie. Big deal!! I don't need them. I am a twelve year old blue-blooded American boy, after all. I pushed the blue button on my converter and, thank God, my Aunt and Uncle disappeared.

My Mom called to me. "Chuck, did you zap Sam and Annie?"

"Yes, Mom."

"What took you so long? You don't think we bought you that contraption for nothing, do you?"

"No Mom."

Part 2

(where in Chuck gets even)

If the world were only mine,
What a wonderful world it would be.
I could influence the world,
And put up a sign that says,
"Please don't pee on me!!"

Part 3

When I was young and still a boy,
The world was bright and life was long.
I thought that I was here to annoy,
All God's creatures with a word or a song.

Now that the world has gotten older,
And all within me has grown stronger,
I see that life is very much colder,
And that life cannot be that much longer.

Part 4

The Present is March 4, 1985. I am now looking for a job or trying to sell my soul for a living. It is 2:20 A.M. No one is awake, not even Jesse, my son. I wish there were words to describe the feelings that I have right now. I feel so much stronger than I ever have before. It is a nice feeling. I also feel very sad that my relationship with my parents has not been a better one. My name is David Samuelson and I am an M.D.; which stands for manic-depressive. What follows this is a journey through the nightmare world of a manic-depressive. The story and poems previously offered are written by me and so is this poem written when I was 12.

> Why do people get depressed?
> There are many reasons, nonetheless.
> Some people lose confidence in themselves.
> Others lose confidence in what they've done.
> Still others lose confidence in their futures.
> These are the uncertainties of life;
> What will happen, has happened and is happening.
> But, the most important thing to know,
> Is the knowledge that life goes on no matter what.
> Sure, life has its ups and downs,
> But, you can't enjoy the good times,
> If you want to end it all when things go bad.
> So, take a tip from someone who knows.
> Enjoy the good life while it's here.
> And when depression starts to reappear.
> Just go out and drink a nice cold beer.

I thought that must be the answer because that is what my father used to do. And everybody knows, "Father Knows Best".

What follows now is not very easy for me to talk about. You see, pain is real and it never really goes away. The depressions that I have experienced over the years, starting when I was about 5 years old, did nothing short of devastating my life. Feelings of inadequacy, of fear; not just mild fear, scared stiff fear. I was afraid of doing anything wrong or of being admonished for breaking any rules. Being depressed, for me, meant being locked in a cold dungeon with no food or water and at the same time suffering from every known disease and ailment that your mind can create. How I hated that. I have come a long way since then. What follows is my life story; filled with documentation and writings done at various times during the last ten years which describe how I felt at the time, better than any words I can add right now. I hope you can learn something from my life. I know I have.

I guess you are wondering why I wrote this book. I am thirty years old, white, male, in good health and of Jewish descent. Well, it's a long story. There are things that happen in everybody's lives that shape them into what they are today. In my case, these happenings are different, peculiar and unusual. I am being redundant you say? I don't think so. My life has been full of surprises and one which I would not change even if I could. I guess I am boring you already so I will get down to the story of my life and my "roots" in life.

I was born in Michael Reese hospital on a rainy day. It was October 5, 1954. I don't remember too much about it except the hearsay that my parents have given me, which isn't too much. Since I can't tell you anything substantial about how I came into this world, let me tell you a little about my parents and sister and, of course, the rest of my illustrious family. Both of my parents were born in West Germany in the mid 20's between the two World Wars. Both of them, as far as I know, were very happy in Germany. They didn't know each other until they came to this country in the late 30's. All you history buffs will remember that was the time that Hitler came to power. You also know that they were very lucky even getting out of Germany alive. They came here in search of a place where they would not be persecuted for being alive. My father's family tried to make it working a farm in Iowa, but they couldn't make a go of it. They both eventually moved to the south side of Chicago in Hyde Park; near the great waters of Lake Michigan.

Both of my parents had a hard time making it in Chicago. They didn't know the language and the Chicagoans didn't want the Germans in their neighborhood. My mother had an especially hard time of it because she was such a sensitive little girl. Every harsh word that was said, to her, hurt her, but she didn't let anybody know that. She would hang around with the "gentile" children and when anybody said anything to her, even if she understood what they said to her, demeaning of course, she would pretend she did not understand it and that made everybody happy, including my mother. But, that started problems which exist to this day. The problem of communication. I will speak more about that later. My father, on the other hand, was different and he knew it. He dressed funny, or so my mother says. The only thing, at that time, that my father could do well was to run faster than the rest of the kids. I wonder why. He went off to fight against the Germans. Anyway, my father apprenticed as a butcher when he was in his late teens and became a very good one. He grew muscles on his body where most people don't even know they exist.

September 29, 1995

03:30 AM

I can't see tomorrow.
I don't want to see today.
The past is my nightmare,
Which I need to put away.

I have to dream about tomorrow,
While wishing today brings a smile.
I have to live down my past;
While forgiveness is out of style.

I have hurt the ones I love,
Not by design, but in pain.
Learning to live has been so hard.
It's left a permanent stain.

I wish I could change the past,
But no one can; it's always there.
Learning from mistakes is tantamount.
If only today could show I care.

Happiness is my goal in life.
It can be done; I see the light.
I'll need all my helping friends,
And the strength to love; not to bite.

Afterword

Oh, I'm on my way I know I am.
Somewhere not so far from here.
All I know is all I feel right now.
I feel the power growing in my hair.
Oh, life is like a maze of doors,
And they all open from the side your on.
Just keep on pushing hard boy, try as you may,
You're going to wind up where you started from!

Cat Stevens

CPSIA information can be obtained
at www.ICGtesting.com
Printed in the USA
FSHW010846211020
74930FS